PET/CT in Gastrointestinal Cancer

Guest Editor

ROLAND HUSTINX, MD, PhD

PET CLINICS

www.pet.theclinics.com

Consulting Editor
ABASS ALAVI, MD, PhD (Hon)

April 2008 • Volume 3 • Number 2

SAUNDERS an imprint of ELSEVIER, Inc.

W.B. SAUNDERS COMPANY
A Division of Elsevier Inc.

1600 John F. Kennedy Boulevard ● Suite 1800 ● Philadelphia, Pennsylvania 19103-2899

http://www.theclinics.com

PET CLINICS Volume 3, Number 2
April 2008 ISSN 1556-8598, ISBN 10: 1-4160-6647-0, ISBN-13: 978-1-4160-6647-7

Editor: Barton Dudlick
Developmental Editor: Theresa Collier

PET Clinics (ISSN 1556-8598) is published quarterly by W.B. Saunders, 360 Park Avenue South, New York, NY 10010-1710. Months of publication are January, April, July, and October. Business and Editorial Offices: 1600 John F. Kennedy Blvd., Suite 1800, Philadelphia, PA 19103-2899. Accounting and Circulation Offices: 11830 Westline Industrial Drive, St. Louis, MO 63146. Periodicals postage paid at New York, NY, and additional mailing offices. Subscription prices per year are $196.00 (US individuals), $274.00 (US institutions), $97.00 (US students), $223.00 (Canadian individuals), $306.00 (Canadian institutions), $118.00 (Canadian students), $237.00 (foreign individuals), $306.00 (foreign institutions), and $118.00 (foreign students). To receive student and resident rate, orders must be accompanied by name of affiliated institution, date of term, and the signature of program/residency coordinator on institution letterhead. Orders will be billed at individual rate until proof of status is received. Foreign air speed delivery is included in all Clinics subscription prices. All prices are subject to change without notice. POSTMASTER: Send address changes to PET Clinics, Elsevier Periodicals Customer Service, 11830 Westline Industrial Drive, St. Louis, MO 63146. **Customer service: 1-800-654-2452 (US). From outside of the United States, call 314-453-7041. Fax: 314-453-5170. E-mail: JournalsCustomerService-usa@elsevier.com (for print support); JournalsOnlineSupport-usa@elsevier.com (for online support).**

Reprints. For copies of 100 or more of articles in this publication, please contact the Commercial Reprints Department, Elsevier Inc., 360 Park Avenue South, New York, NY 10010-1710. Tel.: 212-633-3812; Fax: 212-462-1935; E-mail: reprints@elsevier.com.

Printed in the United States of America.

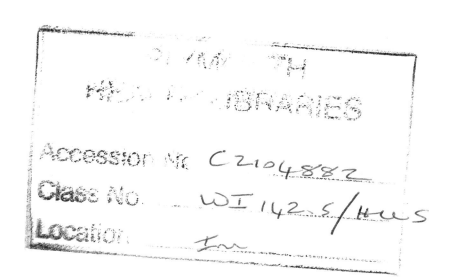

Contributors

CONSULTING EDITOR

ABASS ALAVI, MD, PhD (Hon)
Professor, Division of Nuclear Medicine,
Department of Radiology, Hospital of the
University of Pennsylvania, Philadelphia,
Pennsylvania

GUEST EDITOR

ROLAND HUSTINX, MD, PhD
Chargé de Cours, Division of Nuclear Medicine,
Department of Medical Imaging, University
Hospital of Liège, Campus Universitaire du Sart
Tilman, Liège, Belgium

AUTHORS

ABASS ALAVI, MD, PhD (Hon)
Professor, Division of Nuclear Medicine,
Department of Radiology, Hospital of the
University of Pennsylvania, Philadelphia,
Pennsylvania

VALENTINA AMBROSINI, MD, PhD
Department of Nuclear Medicine, Policlinico S.
Orsola-Malpighi, University of Bologna, Bologna,
Italy

PAOLO CASTELLUCCI, MD
Department of Nuclear Medicine, Policlinico S.
Orsola-Malpighi, University of Bologna, Bologna,
Italy

WICHANA CHAMROONRAT, MD
Department of Radiology, The Children's Hospital
of Philadelphia, Philadelphia, Pennsylvania

DOMINIQUE DELBEKE, MD, PhD, FACNP
Professor and Director, Division of Nuclear
Medicine and PET, Department of Radiology
and Radiological Sciences, Vanderbilt University
Medical Center, Nashville, Tennessee

JASEENA ELIKKOTTIL, MD
Department of Nuclear Medicine, All India Institute
of Medical Sciences, New Delhi, India

JEREMY J. ERASMUS, MBBCh
Professor of Radiology, Department of Diagnostic
Radiology, Division of Diagnostic Imaging, The
University of Texas M. D. Anderson Cancer
Center, Houston, Texas

MEHMET ERTUK, MD
Attending Radiologist, Department of Radiology,
Şişli Etfal Training and Research Hospital, Istanbul,
Turkey

THOMAS F. HANY, MD
Division of Nuclear Medicine, Department
of Medical Radiology, University Hospital,
Raemistrasse, Zurich, Switzerland

KEN HERRMANN, MD
Department of Nuclear Medicine, Klinikum
rechts der Isar, Technische Universität München,
München, Germany

MOHAMED HOUSENI, MD
Department of Radiology, The Children's Hospital
of Philadelphia, Philadelphia, Pennsylvania; and
Department of Radiology, National Liver Institute,
Egypt

ROLAND HUSTINX, MD, PhD
Chargé de Cours, Division of Nuclear Medicine, Department of Medical Imaging, University Hospital of Liège, Campus Universitaire du Sart Tilman, Liège, Belgium

WON JUN KANG, MD, PhD
Assistant Professor of Diagnostic Radiology, Division of Nuclear Medicine, Department of Diagnostic Radiology, Yonsei University College of Medicine, Seodaemun-gu, Seoul, South Korea

RAKESH KUMAR, MD
Associate Professor, Department of Nuclear Medicine, All India Institute of Medical Sciences, New Delhi, India

JONG DOO LEE, MD, PhD
Professor of Diagnostic Radiology, Director of Nuclear Medicine, Division of Nuclear Medicine, Department of Diagnostic Radiology, Yonsei University College of Medicine, Seodaemun-gu, Seoul, South Korea

GEMING LI, MD
Department of Radiology, The Children's Hospital of Philadelphia, Philadelphia, Pennsylvania

MAX LONNEUX, MD, PhD
Professor, Department of Nuclear Medicine, Molecular Imaging and Experimental Radiotherapy Unit, Cliniques Universitaires Saint-Luc, Brussels

WILLIAM H. MARTIN, MD
Associate Professor, Department of Radiology and Radiological Sciences, Vanderbilt University Medical Center, Nashville, Tennessee

GIANCARLO MONTINI, MD
Department of Nuclear Medicine, Policlinico S. Orsola-Malpighi, University of Bologna, Bologna, Italy

ERIC M. ROHREN, MD, PhD
Associate Professor of Nuclear Medicine and Radiology, Department of Nuclear Medicine, Division of Diagnostic Imaging, The University of Texas M. D. Anderson Cancer Center, Houston, Texas

SUHAS SINGLA, MD
Department of Nuclear Medicine, All India Institute of Medical Sciences, New Delhi, India

TINO TANCREDI, MD
Division of Nuclear Medicine, Department of Medical Imaging, University Hospital of Liège, Campus Universitaire du Sart Tilman B, Liège, Belgium

ANNICK D. VAN DEN ABBEELE, MD
Chief, Department of Radiology, Dana-Farber Cancer Institute, Boston; Associate Professor of Radiology, Harvard Medical School, Boston; Founding Director, Center for Biomedical Imaging in Oncology (CBIO), Dana-Farber Cancer Institute, Boston; Co-Director, Tumor Imaging Metrics Core (TIMC), Dana-Farber/Harvard Cancer Center, Boston, Massachusetts

HINRICH A. WIEDER, MD
Department of Radiology, Klinikum rechts der Isar, Technische Universität München, München, Germany

NANCY WITVROUW, MD
Division of Nuclear Medicine, Department of Medical Imaging, University Hospital of Liège, Campus Universitaire du Sart Tilman, Liège, Belgium

MIJIN YUN, MD, PhD
Associate Professor of Diagnostic Radiology, Division of Nuclear Medicine, Department of Diagnostic Radiology, Yonsei University College of Medicine, Seodaemun-gu, Seoul, South Korea

HONGMING ZHUANG, MD, PhD
Department of Radiology, The Children's Hospital of Philadelphia, Philadelphia, Pennsylvania

Contents

> PET/CT methodology is intrinsically divided into PET and CT data acquisition, whereas CT data are used for attenuation correction of PET images. Because CT data are also used for lesion localization, attention has been turned on the optimization of CT protocols using oral and intravenous contrast agents. Using oral as well as intravenous contrast media, no significant qualitative as well as quantitative differences were found in corresponding PET data. Further, use of intravenous contrast enhances the diagnostic performance of integrated PET/CT especially for recurrent colorectal cancer, one of the major indications of PET/CT in gastrointestinal cancer.

> The elderly constitute a significant proportion of patient population in most developed countries, and their numbers are expected to increase in the coming years. The number of clinical applications for PET and PET/CT continue to increase. Like other imaging techniques, there are a large number of variants and artifacts in PET and PET/CT, which can result in false-positive results. Understanding normal age-related changes that can lead to imaging variants and artifacts in structure and function of the human body is very important. This article reviews normal age-related variants and artifacts in the imaging appearance of the gastrointestinal tract.

> Esophageal and gastric cancers are among the leading causes of cancer-related deaths worldwide. Determining stage of disease at presentation is important in the selection of appropriate management. PET and integrated PET/CT are increasingly being used to initially stage patients who have esophageal and gastric cancers. Although PET has a limited role in the evaluation of the primary tumor and in the detection of locoregional nodal metastases, it is important in the detection of distant metastases. This article reviews the role of PET and PET/CT imaging in the diagnosis, initial staging, and detection of recurrent disease in patients who have esophageal and gastric cancers and elucidates the appropriate use of PET and PET/CT in determining the T, N, and M descriptors of the American Joint Commission on Cancer's guidelines for pathologic and clinical staging.

PET Clinics

THE CLINICS ARE NOW AVAILABLE ONLINE!

Access your subscription at:
www.theclinics.com

GOAL STATEMENT

The goal of the *PET Clinics* is to keep practicing radiologists and radiology residents up to date with current clinical practice in positron emission tomography by providing timely articles reviewing the state of the art in patient care.

ACCREDITATION

PET Clinics is planned and implemented in accordance with the Essential Areas and Policies of the Accreditation Council for Continuing Medical Education (ACCME) through the joint sponsorship of the University of Virginia School of Medicine and Elsevier. The University of Virginia School of Medicine is accredited by the ACCME to provide continuing medical education for physicians.

The University of Virginia School of Medicine designates this educational activity for a maximum of 60 *AMA PRA Category 1 Credits*™. Physicians should only claim credit commensurate with the extent of their participation in the activity.

The American Medical Association has determined that physicians not licensed in the US who participate in this CME activity are eligible for *AMA PRA Category 1 Credits*™.

Category 1 credit can be earned by reading the text material, taking the CME examination online at http://www.theclinics.com/home/cme, and completing the evaluation. After taking the test, you will be required to review any and all incorrect answers. Following completion of the test and evaluation, your credit will be awarded and you may print your certificate.

FACULTY DISCLOSURE/CONFLICT OF INTEREST

The University of Virginia School of Medicine, as an ACCME accredited provider, endorses and strives to comply with the Accreditation Council for Continuing Medical Education (ACCME) Standards of Commercial Support, Commonwealth of Virginia statutes, University of Virginia policies and procedures, and associated federal and private regulations and guidelines on the need for disclosure and monitoring of proprietary and financial interests that may affect the scientific integrity and balance of content delivered in continuing medical education activities under our auspices.

The University of Virginia School of Medicine requires that all CME activities accredited through this institution be developed independently and be scientifically rigorous, balanced and objective in the presentation/discussion of its content, theories and practices.

All authors/editors participating in an accredited CME activity are expected to disclose to the readers relevant financial relationships with commercial entities occurring within the past 12 months (such as grants or research support, employee, consultant, stock holder, member of speakers bureau, etc.). The University of Virginia School of Medicine will employ appropriate mechanisms to resolve potential conflicts of interest to maintain the standards of fair and balanced education to the reader. Questions about specific strategies can be directed to the Office of Continuing Medical Education, University of Virginia School of Medicine, Charlottesville, Virginia.

The faculty and staff of the University of Virginia Office of Continuing Medical Education have no financial affiliations to disclose.

The authors/editors listed below have identified no professional or financial affiliations for themselves or their spouse/partner:

Abass Alavi, MD, PhD(Hon) (Consulting Editor); Valentina Ambrosini, MD, PhD; Paolo Castellucci, MD; Wichana Chamroonrat, MD; Barton Dudlick (Acquisitions Editor); Jaseena Elikkottil, MD; Jeremy J. Erasmus, Jr., MD, MBBCh; Sukru Mehmet Erturk, MD; Thomas F. Hany, MD; Ken Herrmann, MD; Mohamad Houseni, MD; Roland Hustinx, MD, PhD (Guest Editor); Won Jun Kang, MD, PhD; Rakesh Kumar, MD; Jong Doo Lee, MD, PhD; Geming Li, MD; Max Lonneux, MD, PhD; William H. Martin, MD; Giancarlo Montini, MD; Patrice Rehm, MD (Test Author); Eric M. Rohren, MD, PhD; Suhas Singla, MD; Tino Tancredi, MD; Annick D. Van den Abbeele, MD; Hinrich A. Wieder, MD; Nancy Witvrouw, MD; Mijin Yun, MD, PhD; and Hongmind Zhuang, MD, PhD.

The authors/editors listed below identified the following professional or financial affiliations for themselves or their spouse/partner:

Dominique Delbeke, MD, PhD, FACNP is a consultant for GE Healthcare and Spectrum Dynamics.

Disclosure of Discussion of Non-FDA Approved Uses for Pharmaceutical Products and/or Medical Devices.

The University of Virginia School of Medicine, as an ACCME provider, requires that all faculty presenters identify and disclose any off-label uses for pharmaceutical and medical device products. The University of Virginia School of Medicine recommends that each physician fully review all the available data on new products or procedures prior to clinical use.

TO ENROLL

To enroll in the PET Clinics Continuing Medical Education program, call customer service at 1-800-654-2452 or visit us online at www.theclinics.com/home/cme. The CME program is available to subscribers for an additional fee of $175.00.

Preface

PET/CT in Gastrointestinal Tumors: Fast Technological Changes Lead to Improved Patient Management

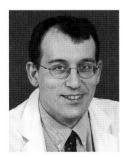

Roland Hustinx, MD, PhD
Guest Editor

Colorectal, stomach, liver, and esophageal cancers rank third, fourth, sixth, and eighth, respectively, in terms of worldwide incidence. Furthermore, liver, esophageal, stomach, and pancreatic cancers figure among the tumors with the highest mortality-to-incidence rate ratios.[1] Gastrointestinal malignancies are thus a major health issue, with an estimated number of new diagnoses close to 3 million worldwide annually. Screening strategies are being designed, and treatments are increasingly effective, especially for colorectal cancer, which is the most common gastrointestinal cancer in the western world. Surgery is proposed to an increasing number of patients with recurrence of colorectal cancer, mostly but not exclusively, in patients with liver metastases. Locoregional treatments, such as radiofrequency ablation, can be used in combination with other modalities, as chemotherapy regimens have been improved as well. In parallel with therapeutic improvements, radiological imaging techniques have evolved tremendously. Multislice CT allow for extremely fast scanning, therefore suppressing all respiratory artifacts and providing high-resolution images of the organs and tissues at the various phases of contrast enhancement. Virtual colonoscopy using a single breath-hold spiral thin-slice CT acquisition after appropriate bowel cleansing generates high-quality 2- and 3-dimensional representations of the entire large bowel.[2] Ultrasonography (US)

with IV contrast agents (microbubbles) show much improved diagnostic performances compared to unenhanced US, especially in the liver. MR imaging has witnessed several major technological advances, with stronger magnetic gradients and improved coils, along with new, liver-specific contrast agents. Finally, PET/CT has become the standard positron imaging procedure, replacing standalone PET, with better crystals and faster electronics. Moreover, the most recent PET/CT devices are equipped with high-end multislice spiral CT, so that full diagnostic CT, including complex procedures such as virtual colonoscopy, can now be combined with FDG imaging.[3] Such dramatic progress in the field of imaging has considerably modified the diagnostic and staging work-up of many cancer diseases, with new diagnostic algorithms being proposed, although the field is changing so rapidly that consensus or widely accepted guidelines are yet to be established in several instances.

MAJOR INDICATIONS OF PET/CT GASTROINTESTINAL CANCERS
Colorectal Cancer

FDG PET/CT is now considered the standard of care for detecting and staging suspected recurrence of colorectal carcinoma. PET has a direct impact on patient management in up to two-thirds

PET Clin 3 (2008) xi–xiii
doi:10.1016/j.cpet.2008.11.001
1556-8598/08/$ – see front matter © 2008 Elsevier Inc. All rights reserved.

of cases.[4] PET/CT is recommended in the preoperative assessment of patients who are candidates for surgical resection of liver metastases.[5] Regarding liver metastases, PET/CT in fact offers the best combination of sensitivity and specificity among all available techniques, with the exception of small subcentimeter lesions, which might be better depicted using MRI with liver-specific contrast enhancement.[6,7] In addition, recent data support using PET as a first-line imaging procedure in the systematic surveillance of high-risk patients,[8] although such an approach remains to be fully validated. Another emerging application is the initial staging of rectal cancers, particularly before multimodal therapies such as neoadjuvant chemo-radiation[9.]

Esophageal and Gastric Cancer

FDG-PET/CT is clearly useful in the initial staging of patients who have esophageal cancers, prior to curative surgical resection. Its role is limited in the evaluation of the primary tumor and in the detection of loco-regional nodal metastases, which are better obtained with endoscopy and echoendoscopy. However, PET imaging is important in the detection of distant metastases. In this regard, PET and PET/CT can spare inappropriate surgical resections, mainly because of the detection of distant metastases not diagnosed by conventional evaluation.[10] Furthermore, there is growing evidence supporting the use of FDG-PET for early evaluation of the response to treatment, whether the treatment is chemotherapy or radiotherapy.[11,12] Similarly, evaluating the metabolic response in order to adapt the treatment scheme appears to be a very promising indication of FDG-PET in gastric cancer.[13] Additionally, in patients with suspected recurrent disease, PET and PET/CT can be helpful to detect sites of metastatic disease.

Cancer of the Pancreas

Although the initially enthusiastic results of FDG-PET imaging have been somewhat tempered by more recent data, it remains useful in selected cases of preoperative diagnosis.[14] This includes in particular, patients who have suspected pancreatic cancer in whom CT fails to identify a discrete tumor mass or in whom fine-needle aspirations are nondiagnostic. FDG-PET imaging has an additional clinical impact in patients who have a proven cancer, especially with regard to the M staging by detecting CT-occult metastatic disease, thus sparing unnecessary nontherapeutic surgeries.[15] FDG-PET can differentiate between post-therapy changes and recurrence of tumors which are often similar, and is being investigated as a tool for monitoring neo-adjuvant chemo-radiation therapy, with promising results.[16] Despite reasonably good diagnostic performances, PET has not produced a significant impact on management of periampullary carcinomas.[17]

Primary Tumors of the Liver

FDG-PET has shown a poor sensitivity for detecting primary intrahepatic low grade hepatocellular carcinomas (HCC). This does not mean, however, that the technique is useless in this setting. Indeed, increased FDG uptake within tumors may well be a surrogate marker of aggressive behavior and poor clinical outcome in HCCs. Furthermore, FDG-PET appears to be more sensitive for detecting extrahepatic metastases and therefore useful in the pretherapeutic staging of HCCs.[18] Fatty acid metabolism is another target available for molecular imaging, and it is very possible that using dual tracer approaches, FDG and C11-acetate for instance, might be of great help in selecting patients for surgery, thanks to a very high negative predictive value.[19] FDG-PET and PET/CT are useful in staging, prediction of prognosis, evaluation of recurrence, and treatment response in cholangiocarcinomas with the notable exception of periductal-infiltrating cholangiocarcinomas.[20,21]

Neuroendocrine Tumors

Although neuroendocrine tumors are infrequent, this is a very exciting field of nuclear medicine. Except for poorly differentiated subtypes, the role of FDG-PET is very limited in the evaluation of neuroendocrine tumors.[22] Recently, however, various somatostatine analogues such as DOTA-NOC and DOTA-TOC, have been labeled with the generator-produced ^{68}Ga. The combined PET/CT modality using these highly specific compounds has shown extremely encouraging results that are significantly better than the classical monophotonic scintigraphy.[23,24] F-DOPA is another potentially useful compound, but it is not clear whether it will prove useful in comparison with the somatostatine analogues.[24] In any case, there is a whole new field of investigation lying ahead, with the advantage of using tracers that can be widely available at a reasonable cost.

Roland Hustinx, MD, PhD
Division of Nuclear Medicine
University Hospital of Liège
Campus Universitaire du Sart Tilman B35
4000 Liège, Belgium

E-mail address:
rhustinx@chu.ulg.ac.be (R. Hustinx)

REFERENCES

1. Kamangar F, Dores GM, Anderson WF. Patterns of cancer incidence, mortality, and prevalence across five continents: defining priorities to reduce cancer disparities in different geographic regions of the world. J Clin Oncol 2006;24(14):2137–50.
2. Hoeffel C, Mulé S, Romaniuk B, et al. Advances in radiological imaging of gastrointestinal tumors. Crit Rev Oncol Hematol 2008 Jul 30 [Epub ahead of print].
3. Veit P, Kühle C, Beyer T, et al. Whole body positron emission tomography/computed tomography (PET/CT) tumour staging with integrated PET/CT colonography: technical feasibility and first experiences in patients with colorectal cancer. Gut 2006;55(1):68–73.
4. Scott AM, Gunawardana DH, Kelley B, et al. PET Changes Management and Improves Prognostic Stratification in Patients with Recurrent Colorectal Cancer: Results of a Multicenter Prospective Study. J Nucl Med 2008;49(9):1451–7.
5. Wiering B, Krabbe PF, Dekker HM, et al. The role of FDG-PET in the selection of patients with colorectal liver metastases. Ann Surg Oncol 2007;14(2):771–9.
6. Chua SC, Groves AM, Kayani I, et al. The impact of 18F-FDG PET/CT in patients with liver metastases. Eur J Nucl Med Mol Imaging 2007;34(12):1906–14.
7. Kong G, Jackson C, Koh DM, et al. The use of 18F-FDG PET/CT in colorectal liver metastases-comparison with CT and liver MRI. Eur J Nucl Med Mol Imaging 2008;35(7):1323–9.
8. Sobhani I, Tiret E, Lebtahi R, et al. Early detection of recurrence by 18FDG-PET in the follow-up of patients with colorectal cancer. Br J Cancer 2008; 98(5):875–80.
9. Davey K, Heriot AG, Mackay J, et al. The impact of 18-fluorodeoxyglucose positron emission tomography-computed tomography on the staging and management of primary rectal cancer. Dis Colon Rectum 2008;51(7):997–1003.
10. Meyers BF, Downey RJ, Decker PA, et al. The utility of positron emission tomography in staging of potentially operable carcinoma of the thoracic esophagus: results of the American College of Surgeons Oncology Group Z0060 trial. J Thorac Cardiovasc Surg 2007;133(3):738–45.
11. Lordick F, Ott K, Krause BJ, et al. PET to assess early metabolic response and to guide treatment of adenocarcinoma of the oesophagogastric junction: the MUNICON phase II trial. Lancet Oncol 2007; 8(9):797–805.
12. Wieder HA, Brücher BL, Zimmermann F, et al. Time course of tumor metabolic activity during chemoradiotherapy of esophageal squamous cell carcinoma and response to treatment. J Clin Oncol 2004;22(5): 900–8.
13. Ott K, Herrmann K, Lordick F, et al. Early metabolic response evaluation by fluorine-18 fluorodeoxyglucose positron emission tomography allows in vivo testing of chemosensitivity in gastric cancer: long-term results of a prospective study. Clin Cancer Res 2008;14(7):2012–8.
14. Pakzad F, Groves AM, Ell PJ. The role of positron emission tomography in the management of pancreatic cancer. Semin Nucl Med 2006;36(3):248–56.
15. Rose DM, Delbeke D, Beauchamp RD, et al. 18Fluorodeoxyglucose-positron emission tomography in the management of patients with suspected pancreatic cancer. Ann Surg 1999;229(5):729–37 discussion 737–8.
16. Ruf J, Lopez Hänninen E, Oettle H, et al. Detection of recurrent pancreatic cancer: comparison of FDG-PET with CT/MRI. Pancreatology 2005;5(2-3): 266–72.
17. Kalady MF, Clary BM, Clark LA, et al. Clinical utility of positron emission tomography in the diagnosis and management of periampullary neoplasms. Ann Surg Oncol 2002;9(8):799–806.
18. Yoon KT, Kim JK, Kim do Y, et al. Role of 18F-fluorodeoxyglucose positron emission tomography in detecting extrahepatic metastasis in pretreatment staging of hepatocellular carcinoma. Oncology 2007;72(Suppl 1):104–10.
19. Ho CL, Chen S, Yeung DW, et al. Dual-tracer PET/CT imaging in evaluation of metastatic hepatocellular carcinoma. J Nucl Med 2007;48(6):902–9.
20. Corvera CU, Blumgart LH, Akhurst T, et al. 18F-fluorodeoxyglucose positron emission tomography influences management decisions in patients with biliary cancer. J Am Coll Surg 2008;206(1):57–65.
21. Moon CM, Bang S, Chung JB, et al. Usefulness of 18F-fluorodeoxyglucose positron emission tomography in differential diagnosis and staging of cholangiocarcinomas. J Gastroenterol Hepatol 2008; 23(5):759–65.
22. Pasquali C, Rubello D, Sperti C, et al. Neuroendocrine tumor imaging: can 18F-fluorodeoxyglucose positron emission tomography detect tumors with poor prognosis and aggressive behavior? World J Surg 1998;22(6):588–92.
23. Kowalski J, Henze M, Schuhmacher J, et al. Evaluation of positron emission tomography imaging using [68Ga]-DOTA-D Phe(1)-Tyr(3)-Octreotide in comparison to [111In]-DTPAOC SPECT. First results in patients with neuroendocrine tumors. Mol Imaging Biol 2003;5(1):42–8.
24. Ambrosini V, Tomassetti P, Castellucci P, et al. Comparison between 68Ga-DOTA-NOC and 18F-DOPA PET for the detection of gastro-entero-pancreatic and lung neuro-endocrine tumours. Eur J Nucl Med Mol Imaging 2008;35(8):1431–8.

PET/CT in Gastrointestinal Cancer: Methodological Aspects

Thomas F. Hany, MD

KEYWORDS

• PET/CT • FDG • Contrast agents • Gastrointestinal cancers

Anatomic information is an additional benefit in co-registered PET/CT imaging and improves localization of pathologic fluorodeoxyglucose (FDG) uptake.[1,2] This information is generated from axial low-dose CT images. Different CT systems (single- or multi-slice spiral CT scanner) are used in the hybrid PET/CT system.[3,4] Because the application of contrast media is a standard procedure in CT, application of contrast has also been mandated in co-registered imaging.[5] For abdominal malignancies, single- up to triple-phase intravenous contrast-enhanced CT protocols including arterial, portal-venous, and late-phase imaging are implemented depending on the tumor type.[6] Especially in the evaluation of the liver in primary liver tumors like hepatocellular carcinoma or metastases from neuroendocrine carcinoma of the gastrointestinal tract (GIT), as well as in the evaluation of pancreatic cancer, arterial phase imaging is a standard procedure.[7] Additionally, according to the evaluated disease, positive or negative oral contrasts are given.

The effect of positive contrast agents generally used in radiological procedures is based on increased attenuation of the x-ray beam and therefore increased density values in CT images. Oral contrast agents are used for delineation of the GIT from adjacent structures. Here, the optimal intestinal contrast in the entire GIT is obtained not before 45 to 60 minutes after ingestion of positive oral contrast. Intravenously injected contrast agents are used to delineate the gross vascular anatomy, meanwhile dynamic scanning allows for the evaluation of organ structures owing to their characteristic pattern of enhancement. Optimal contrast is reached several seconds to minutes after the application. Depending on the scanner used (single-slice vs. multi-slice scanner), different injection protocols are used.[6] Water as a low-density contrast agent has been used with variable success in imaging of the stomach as well as the rectum.[8] Recently, liquid low-density oral contrast agents as a mixture of locust bean gum and mannitol for CT have been demonstrated to be favorable in the use for PET/CT.[9]

Technical issues, indications, and implications in the use of positive as well as negative oral contrast agents and intravenous contrast enhancement in PET/CT imaging are discussed.

TECHNICAL ISSUES RELATED TO PET IMAGING

Not only different do crystal materials used for photon detection but also two different data acquisition modes for emission scanning followed by various image reconstruction algorithms complicate the comparison of the available PET/CT scanner systems. Lutetium (LSO, LYSO)–Germanium (GSO) as well as Bismutgermanate (BGO)-based crystals are used in different scanner types.[10–12] PET-emission data are acquired in two-dimensional (2D) as well as in 3D mode, albeit the 3D mode seems to be the preferential method.[12,13] Additionally, different new reconstruction algorithms are used to improve image quality.[13]

CT data are foremost used for attenuation correction and as anatomic reference frame in PET/CT. The measured attenuation maps in PET/CT are the CT images obtained from polychromatic radiographs of around 100 keV. These are transformed to μ-maps at the spatial resolution

Division of Nuclear Medicine, Department of Medical Radiology, University Hospital, Raemistrasse 100, CH-8091 Zurich, Switzerland
E-mail address: thomas.hany@usz.ch

PET Clin 3 (2008) 115–122
doi:10.1016/j.cpet.2008.08.006
1556-8598/08/$ – see front matter © 2008 Elsevier Inc. All rights reserved.

corresponding to the PET images, and correspond to attenuation images at 511 keV, the photon energy relevant in PET. It turns out that this transformation is relatively simple and can be achieved by a bi-linear lookup table with its inflection point at 0 Hounsfield units (HU).[14] The artifacts that can be generated in PET images owing to the use of CT data transformed into μ-maps are related to the accumulation of highly concentrated CT contrast agents, CT beam hardening artifacts as a result of metallic implants, and physiologic motion. Additionally, major artifacts occur in the regions adjacent to the heart and the diaphragm including the liver. Specifically, PET data are acquired most frequently during free breathing, which corresponds largely to an end-expiratory position of the diaphragm, while CT is normally acquired at maximum inspiration. This leads to an anatomic mismatch between the two data sets with the lungs more expanded in CT. An analysis of this problem has shown that with the modern fast CT scanners it is probably best to also acquire the CT data during tidal breathing. Ideally, the CT data are acquired during end expiration, but frequently patient cooperation is problematic to achieve this.[15] Another approach is to use respiratory gated 4D-PET/CT, which probably has not only an advantage in lung but also in upper abdominal imaging including the liver.[16]

ORAL CONTRAST AGENTS

Iodinated oral contrast agents as well as barium sulfate are routinely used as orally administered dilute contrast materials in CT imaging. Gastrografin (Schering AG, Berlin, Germany) is a water-soluble neutral iodinated contrast medium and mostly used in patients with suspicion of possible leakage into the intraperitoneal space. The application of Gastrografin can lead to accelerated emptying of the GIT. The other mainly used oral contrast agent is a barium sulfate–containing solution, mostly used in patients without history of abdominal problems since leakage into the intraperitoneal space can lead to life-threatening peritonitis.

Oral contrast agents have to be dissolved by water to an amount of 1 liter and are given 45 minutes before CT scanning to obtain optimal contrast of the entire GIT. Side effects of both compounds are mild (gastrointestinal discomfort, diarrhea, constipation) and only temporary. To obtain optimal contrast also of the stomach, a last sip of contrast solution is taken just before patient positioning on the table.

Clinical studies analyzed contrast agent distribution in CT images of PET/CT studies using oral contrast agent and the correlation with FDG uptake as well as localization of FDG uptake and possible introduction of artifacts. Visual image analysis revealed no significant difference in FDG uptake in PET images regarding the GIT except the ascending colon. It is most unlikely that increased FDG uptake observed in standard PET scans is attributable to peristalsis-induced increased muscular uptake, because in this case all regions would have been affected. A possible explanation of increased FDG uptake in the ascending colon may be a result of physiologic causes like intestinal secretion of FDG-containing fluid induced by administration of Gastrografin. However, this slight increase in FDG accumulation does not interfere with diagnosis. No correlation was found in the location of increased FDG uptake and contrast media in the CT images. This is because CT data are acquired first, whereas the emission data take place between 2 and 10 minutes later. In the meantime, contrast agent is traveling farther through the gastrointestinal system.[17] Further, calculated standard uptake values (SUV) in the reconstructed PET images showed only small differences, in the range of 1% to 2%. Therefore, no significant quantitative error is introduced when using normally diluted positive contrast media.[18] Nondiluted intravenous or impacted positive oral contrast agent with very high HU units, however, may introduce artifacts similar to metallic prosthesis.

Recently, liquid low-density oral contrast agents as a mixture of locust bean gum and mannitol for CT have been demonstrated to be favorable in the use for PET/CT.[9] Intestinal uptake seems to be less seen compared with positive contrast agents. This type of contrast agent is commercially available in the United States but not yet in Europe. Also, milk as a liquid low-density oral contrast agent has proven to be cost-effective and easy to use, however it cannot be used in PET/CT imaging for obvious reasons regarding fasting.[19] Concluding from the available data, oral positive as well as negative contrast agents can be used in PET/CT imaging without introducing artifacts in PET images. However, when PET/CT data are used for radiation treatment planning, oral contrast media have to be omitted owing to interference with needed densitometry in the field of radiation.

DISEASE-SPECIFIC INDICATIONS REGARDING ORAL CONTRAST AGENTS
Negative Oral Contrast Agents

As mentioned previously, potable water can be used as a simple and highly cost-effective oral contrast agent. Ingestion of 1 liter of water is started approximately 45 minutes before PET/CT during a period of 20 to 30 minutes. The last sip of water is taken just before patient positioning on the table.

Major indications are the following:

1. primary staging and restaging of stomach cancer, as water distension allows the evaluation of the gastric wall
2. primary staging and restaging of pancreatic cancer, as positive contrast agent hampers the evaluation of the pancreatic head owing to possible artifacts
3. primary staging and restaging of neuroendocrine tumors of the GIT (in conjunction with F18-DOPA or Ga68- DOTA-TOC PET/CT imaging)

Positive Oral Contrast Agents

Positive oral contrast agents are used for all abdominal malignancies otherwise not mentioned above. Ingestion of 1 liter of contrast solution is started approximately 45 minutes before PET/CT during a period of 20 to 30 minutes. In patients with history of lung aspiration, oral contrast agent containing barium sulfate should be used. For patients with possible leakage/fistula into the abdominal cavity/peritoneum, iodinated oral contrast agent should be used (eg, Gastrographin). A last sip of contrast solution is taken just before patient positioning on the table.

INTRAVENOUS CONTRAST MEDIA

Mostly, iodinated non-ionic contrast media with different available concentrations of iodine with a favorable safety profile are used for intravenous applications. However, specific allergic reactions to iodine and induction of renal insufficiency have to be kept in mind when performing contrast-enhanced CT.[20]

With the fast technical development in CT technology, data acquisition speed has been accelerated significantly when comparing single-slice spiral to multi-slice spiral technology. One of the main developments was the introduction of multi-row detectors and increased rotation speed of the gantry system. Coverage of the entire thorax and abdomen when using a multi-slice spiral CT scanner can be acquired within less than 30 seconds compared to more than 80 seconds with an advanced single-slice spiral technology. Injection protocols had to be adapted to shorter data acquisition times, whereas the total dose of contrast media could favorably be reduced.[6] Therefore, injection protocols are strongly dependent on the used CT hardware. These circumstances have influenced the application of iodinated contrast to a certain point in co-registered PET/CT.

Two different approaches for the use of intravenous contrast have been introduced. In a single-step approach, contrast is given during the acquisition of CT data used for attenuation correction and no further CT scanning is needed.[5] The other approach includes two CT data acquisitions. One fast, whole-body low-dose CT for attenuation correction (AC), and an additional dedicated contrast-enhanced CT in the region of interest after completion of the PET/CT exam if necessary.[21]

Performing a dedicated contrast-enhanced single- to multi-phase CT data acquisition after completion of PET/CT in a defined anatomic region has two advantages. First, in cases with extended disease or normal findings, the contrast injection may be unnecessary. Second, the possibility of acquiring a multi-phase, contrast-enhanced CT during the arterial, venous, and parenchymal phases is more efficient compared with a single phase acquisition.[22] Therefore, a comprehensive diagnostic workup in a single session can be achieved.

INTRAVENOUS CONTRAST AGENTS

Arterial phase imaging (fixed delay imaging: scan starts 30 to 40 seconds after start of contrast medium injection or use of a bolus triggering technique); an additional portal-venous phase is acquired routinely.

1. hepatocellular carcinoma
2. cholangio carcinoma (**Fig. 1A–D**)
3. pancreatic cancer
4. neuroendocrine cancer of the GIT
5. any indication in which evaluation of arterial vasculature is necessary

In portal-venous phase imaging, the scan starts 60 to 70 seconds after start of injection. Delineation of portal-venous system and hepatic veins is needed for correct segmental localization of liver lesions. There is differentiation between malignant and benign lesions (eg, hemangioma). The following are indications for portal-venous phase imaging only:

1. colorectal cancer
2. gastrointestinal stroma tumor (GIST)
3. evaluation of liver metastases from non-GI tumors

DISCUSSION

From a technical point of view, intravenous as well as oral contrast-enhanced CT can be used for attenuation correction in PET/CT imaging without subjective or objective degradation of PET images in the abdomen.

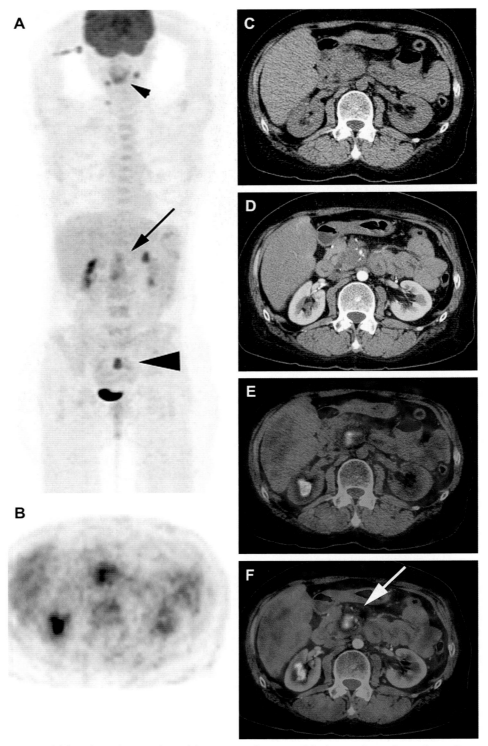

Fig. 1. A 56-year-old female patient evaluated for pancreatic cancer (*black arrow*): maximum-intensity projection PET image (*A*), axial PET (*B*), non-enhanced CT (*C*), arterial phase-contrast–enhanced CT (*D*), and fused non-enhanced (*E*) and contrast-enhanced PET/CT (*F*) at the level of the pancreas. Only contrast-enhanced PET/CT allows reliable determination of the encasement of the mesenteric artery by the pancreatic cancer (*white arrow*). Base of the tongue (*small black arrowhead*) and rectal cancer (*large black arrowhead*) were found incidentally (see *A*).

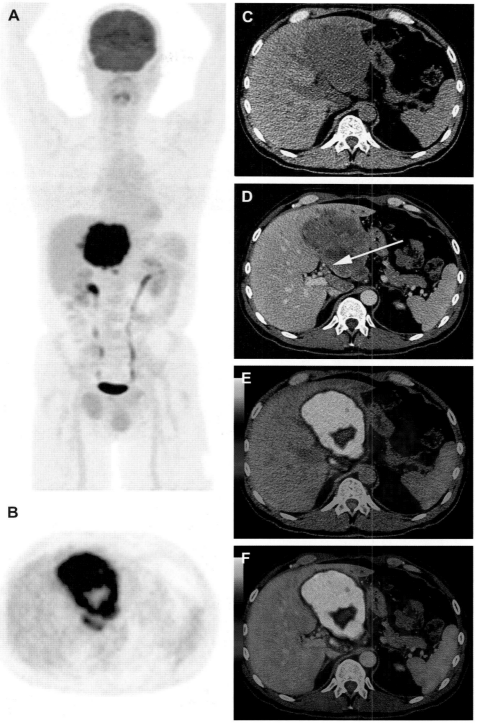

Fig. 2. A 42-year-old male patient evaluated for cholangio-carcinoma of the left liver lobe: maximum-intensity projection PET image (*A*), axial PET (*B*), non-enhanced CT (*C*), portal-venous phase-contrast–enhanced CT (*D*), and fused non-enhanced (*E*) and contrast-enhanced PET/CT (*F*) at the level of the left portal vein. Besides portal lymph node involvement, occlusion of the left portal vein is demonstrated (*white arrow* in *D*).

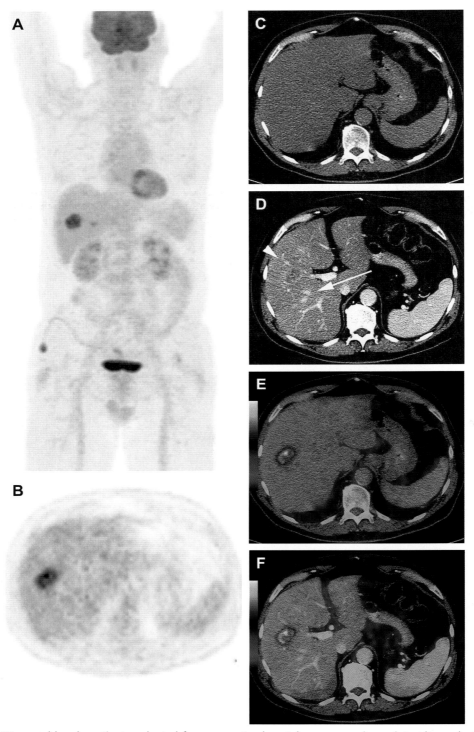

Fig. 3. A 64-year-old male patient evaluated for recurrent colorectal cancer: maximum-intensity projection PET image (*A*), axial PET (*B*), non-enhanced CT (*C*), portal-venous phase-contrast–enhanced CT (*D*), and fused non-enhanced (*E*) and contrast-enhanced PET/CT (*F*) at the level of the left portal vein. The liver metastasis in liver segment V can only reliably be assigned to the segment with the clear delineation of the right (*white arrow*) and middle (*white arrowhead*) hepatic vein (see image *D*). A second metastasis in liver segment IVB is not displayed on the axial images.

From a clinical point of view, several approaches have been used to evaluate the added value of contrast enhancement in PET/CT. Essentially, additional benefit of integrated contrast-enhanced CT seems to be logical but data regarding diagnostic efficacy or even cost-effectiveness is only sparse. Basically, if any knowledge regarding vascular structures is needed, a contrast-enhanced CT seems to be necessary. For example, in pancreatic cancer, not only distant metastases are precluding a curative approach by surgery but also delineation of arterial vascular involvement of the celiac trunk and mesenteric artery (**Fig. 1**A–F). Further, portal vein involvement mainly by primary liver tumors like cholangiocarcinoma is most important for planning a surgical procedure (**Fig. 2**A–F). Arterial as well as portal-venous phase CT imaging is warranted for the above-mentioned indications and indeed can be integrated into the PET/CT protocol. Whenever the PET/CT study is used to evaluate a certain disease for the presence of distant metastases, a routine contrast-enhanced study has to be applied in the light of the prevalence of disease, because in many cases, contrast enhancement will not be necessary. For example, contrast-enhanced CT of the brain and neck is unlikely necessary in the evaluation of a patient with colon cancer. Therefore, a tailored contrast-enhanced PET/CT protocol for each indication seems to be the most effective approach and has to be decided after acquisition of PET data on-site. For certain indications like lymphoma in general, contrast enhancement is probably not needed in the patient follow-up.[23] On the other hand, evaluation of recurrent colorectal carcinoma or presurgical evaluation before liver surgery will definitely need intravenous contrast enhancement. Soyka and colleagues[24] compared contrast-enhanced CT to non-enhanced PET/CT as well as contrast-enhanced PET/CT in restaging of patients with colorectal cancer. The most important advantage of intravenous enhancement integrated into PET/CT was not only the more reliable segmental localization of liver lesions but also a higher confidence in diagnostic accuracy compared with the contrast-enhanced CT alone (**Fig. 3**A–F). The authors therefore concluded that in patients with suspicion or evident recurrent disease, contrast-enhanced PET/CT should be used as the first-line imaging tool.

All of the above-mentioned considerations are made under ideal conditions. To date, patients will arrive with recent imaging studies before they will undergo PET/CT. Therefore, intrinsic limitations do not allow imaging of patients within an appropriate imaging protocol including the use of a multiphase contrast-enhanced CT of selected regions, even though it would be beneficial for the PET/CT imaging study.

All these limitations have to be overcome by a further integration of morphologic and functional imaging modalities and mentalities as well as changes in certain diagnostic paradigms through intensive discussions with our clinical colleagues.

SUMMARY

Intravenous as well as oral contrast-enhanced CT can be used for used for attenuation correction in PET/CT imaging without subjective or objective degradation of PET images in the abdomen. Use of positive as well as negative oral contrast should be encouraged since obvious diagnostic benefit is obtained without harming image quality or the patient. Routine use of intravenous contrast in PET/CT is questionable and has to be further elaborated for each tumor indication of PET/CT imaging. However, for certain indications like recurrent colorectal cancer, a certain level of evidence is available regarding improved diagnostic accuracy of PET/CT imaging.

REFERENCES

1. Kluetz PG, Meltzer CC, Villemagne VL, et al. Combined PET/CT imaging in oncology. Impact on patient management. Clin Positron Imaging 2000;3: 223–30.
2. Townsend DW. A combined PET/CT scanner: the choices. J Nucl Med 2001;42:533–4.
3. Beyer T, Townsend DW, Brun T, et al. A combined PET/CT scanner for clinical oncology. J Nucl Med 2000;41:1369–79.
4. Hany TF, Steinert HC, Goerres GW, et al. PET diagnostic accuracy: improvement with in-line PET-CT system: initial results. Radiology 2002;225:575–81.
5. Antoch G, Saoudi N, Kuehl H, et al. Accuracy of whole-body dual-modality Fluorine-18-2-Fluoro-2-Deoxy-D-Glucose Positron Emission Tomography and Computed Tomography (FDG-PET/CT) for tumor staging in solid tumors: comparison with CT and PET. J Clin Oncol 2004;22:4357–68.
6. Brink JA. Contrast optimization and scan timing for single and multidetector-row computed tomography. J Comput Assist Tomogr 2003;27(Suppl 1):S3–8.
7. Kondo H, Kanematsu M, Goshima S, et al. MDCT of the pancreas: optimizing scanning delay with a bolus-tracking technique for pancreatic, peripancreatic vascular, and hepatic contrast enhancement. AJR Am J Roentgenol 2007;188:751–6.
8. Rossi M, Broglia L, Graziano P, et al. Local invasion of gastric cancer: CT findings and pathologic correlation using 5-mm incremental scanning, hypotonia,

and water filling. AJR Am J Roentgenol 1999;172: 383–8.

9. Antoch G, Kuehl H, Kanja J, et al. Dual-modality PET/CT scanning with negative oral contrast agent to avoid artifacts: introduction and evaluation. Radiology 2004;230:879–85.

10. Antoch G, Stattaus J, Nemat AT, et al. Non-small cell lung cancer: dual-modality PET/CT in preoperative staging. Radiology 2003;229:526–33.

11. Kemp BJ, Kim C, Williams JJ, et al. NEMA NU 2-2001 performance measurements of an LYSO-based PET/CT system in 2D and 3D acquisition modes. J Nucl Med 2006;47:1960–7.

12. Surti S, Kuhn A, Werner ME, et al. Performance of Philips Gemini TF PET/CT scanner with special consideration for its time-of-flight imaging capabilities. J Nucl Med 2007;48:471–80.

13. Strobel K, Rudy M, Treyer V, et al. Objective and subjective comparison of standard 2-D and fully 3-D reconstructed data on a PET/CT system. Nucl Med Commun 2007;28:555–9.

14. Burger C, Goerres G, Schoenes S, et al. PET attenuation coefficients from CT images: experimental evaluation of the transformation of CT into PET 511-keV attenuation coefficients. Eur J Nucl Med Mol Imaging 2002;29:922–7.

15. Goerres GW, Burger C, Kamel E, et al. Respiration-induced attenuation artifact at PET/CT: technical considerations. Radiology 2003;226:906–10.

16. Nehmeh SA, Erdi YE, Pan T, et al. Quantitation of respiratory motion during 4D-PET/CT acquisition. Med Phys 2004;31:1333–8.

17. Dizendorf EV, Treyer V, Von Schulthess GK, et al. Application of oral contrast media in coregistered positron emission tomography-CT. AJR Am J Roentgenol 2002;179:477–81.

18. Dizendorf E, Hany TF, Buck A, et al. Cause and magnitude of the error induced by oral CT contrast agent in CT-based attenuation correction of PET emission studies. J Nucl Med 2003;44:732–8.

19. Koo CW, Shah-Patel LR, Baer JW, et al. Cost-effectiveness and patient tolerance of low-attenuation oral contrast material: milk versus VoLumen. AJR Am J Roentgenol 2008;190:1307–13.

20. Cochran ST, Bomyea K, Sayre JW. Trends in adverse events after IV administration of contrast media. AJR Am J Roentgenol 2001;176:1385–8.

21. Pfannenberg AC, Aschoff P, Brechtel K, et al. Value of contrast-enhanced multiphase CT in combined PET/CT protocols for oncological imaging. Br J Radiol 2007;80:437–45.

22. Keogan MT, McDermott VG, Paulson EK, et al. Pancreatic malignancy: effect of dual-phase helical CT in tumor detection and vascular opacification. Radiology 1997;205:513–8.

23. Schaefer NG, Hany TF, Taverna C, et al. Non-Hodgkin lymphoma and Hodgkin disease: coregistered FDG PET and CT at staging and restaging–do we need contrast-enhanced CT? Radiology 2004;232: 823–9.

24. Soyka JD, Veit-Haibach P, Strobel K, et al. Staging pathways in recurrent colorectal carcinoma: is contrast-enhanced 18F-FDG PET/CT the diagnostic tool of choice? J Nucl Med 2008;49:354–61.

Normal Variants and Effects of Aging on the Gastrointestinal Tract

Rakesh Kumar, MD[a],*, Jaseena Elikkottil, MD[a],
Suhas Singla, MD[a], Abass Alavi, MD, PhD (Hon)[b]

KEYWORDS

- Fluoro-2-deoxy-glucose (FDG) • PET • PET/CT
- Normal variants • Gastrointestinal imaging
- Effects of aging

Age-related spending which mainly include health care costs is projected to increase from 11.2% to 16.7% by 2050 in United States.[1] The causes and basic effects of normal aging on our body is still relatively unknown. Tietz and colleagues[2] contend that more research is necessary to set reference values for interpreting medical information related to older individuals. The changes associated with normal age may be misinterpreted as abnormal if compared with reference values derived from younger populations of individuals. Some studies have also evaluated the changes in organ structure with age.

CT and MRI have been previously established as accurate means of measuring hepatic volume in both pediatric and adult populations.[3–6] Evaluation of tissue function has been largely ignored in past studies. Positron emission tomography (PET) alone and PET- computed tomography (PET-CT) is well established diagnostic imaging technique used for diagnosis, staging and restaging after treatment or recurrence of various cancers.[7–9] The number of clinical applications for PET and PET-CT, therefore continue to increase. In addition, there is growth in the number of PET and PET-CT centers as this technology is becoming affordable. Florine18-fluoro-2-deoxy-D-glucose (FDG) is most commonly used PET radiopharmaceutical, which is an analog of glucose detects the difference in glucose metabolism. However, FDG is not a tumor specific, and an increased uptake may be seen in many benign conditions. Like other diagnostic imaging techniques, there are large number of variants and artifacts. Recently, our group published a study involving large number of patients to assess changes in organ metabolism with age using FDG-PET.[10]

Understanding of these normal age-related changes, which can lead to imaging variants and artifacts in structure and function of the human body, is very important. In the present study we review normal age-related variants and artifacts in the imaging appearance of the gastrointestinal tract. In the present review we divided gastrointestinal system in to two parts: hollow gastrointestinal system (esophagus, stomach, small and large intestines) and solid organs (liver, spleen, and pancreas).

ESOPHAGUS

Normally we do not observe any FDG activity in the esophagus. However, mild diffuse esophageal uptake is often normal variant. This mild diffuse activity is because of some contraction of esophageal smooth muscle. Intense diffuse activity in esophagus is usually associated with benign causes like esophagitis, Barrett's mucosa, post radiation therapy to the thorax, esophageal spasm,

a Department of Nuclear Medicine, All India Institute of Medical Sciences, New Delhi 110029, India
b Division of Nuclear Medicine, Department of Radiology, Hospital of the University of Pennsylvania, Philadelphia, PA, USA
* Corresponding author.
E-mail address: rkphulia@yahoo.com (R. Kumar).

PET Clin 3 (2008) 123–134
doi:10.1016/j.cpet.2008.10.003
1556-8598/08/$ – see front matter © 2008 Elsevier Inc. All rights reserved.

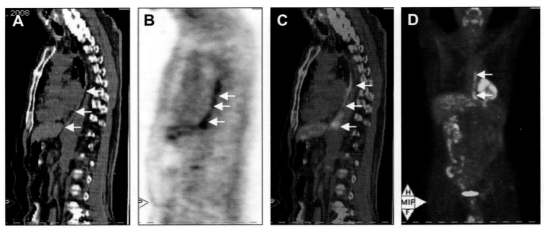

Fig. 1. (*A–D*) Sagittal section of CT, PET, PET-CT, and projection images showing increase FDG uptake in lower half of the esophagus (*arrows*). Patient had received radiotherapy in the chest.

gastrointestinal reflux etc. (**Fig. 1**). Mild to moderate focal FDG uptake is commonly noted at gastroesophageal (GE) junction, which is a normal variant (**Fig. 2**). However, intense FDG uptake at GE junction is associated with esophageal cancer and spasm of GE junction. In some cases, brown fat FDG uptake azygoesophageal recess near GE junction can also be very intense, which can mimic focal uptake in esophagus (**Fig. 3**). PET-CT is very useful to differentiate, if intense focal uptake is due to malignant pathology or due to brown fat. There is circumferential wall thickening and proximal dilatation in cases of cancer while esophagus, structure remains normal if high uptake is due to brown fat. In addition, brown fat FDG uptake can be noted in other body regions and usually appear as bilateral symmetric.

Comparison of the upper esophageal sphincter function of neonates to those of middle-aged adults shows higher sphincter pressure, larger pressure gradient with relaxation and lesser relaxation time in adults. As such, the amount of time that the upper esophageal sphincter remains open during swallowing appears to decrease between infancy and adulthood. In adults, older individuals had decreased resting upper esophageal sphincter pressure and greater delay in relaxation of the sphincter, after contraction, than did younger subjects.[11,12] Similarly, the lower esophageal sphincter and secondary esophageal peristalsis of older adults functions poorly.[12–14] This may point to a weakening of esophageal smooth muscle with age.

STOMACH

Mild to moderate FDG uptake is normal variant in stomach wall, especially when stomach is not dilated with neutral contrast (**Fig. 4**). In some cases there can be intense FDG uptake in stomach. This intense FDG uptake is not necessarily associated with malignancy, but can be seen in benign disease like gastritis, gastroesophageal reflux disease (GERD), pull up stomach surgery, hiatus hernia etc. A maximum normal gastroesophageal SUV of 4.0 was identified by a PET study on a population with a mean age of 57.4 years.[15] Without a specific history of esophagogastric disease, it

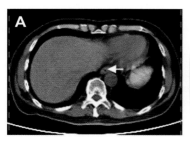
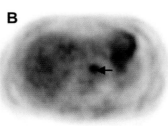
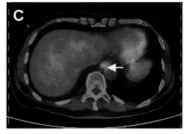

Fig. 2. (*A–C*) Axial section of CT, PET, and PET-CT images showing increase FDG uptake at gastroesophageal junction (*arrow*).

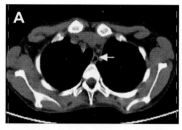 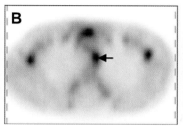 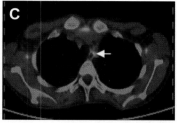

Fig. 3. (A–C) Axial section of CT, PET, and PET-CT images showing increase FDG uptake in brown fat, which appears to be in the wall of esophagus (*arrow*). Note FDG uptake in bilateral axilla and strenal region.

was found not to be associated with neoplasia. Patients with a history of GERD had a slightly higher but not statistically significant SUV peak in the stomach and particularly in the GE junction. Another PET study found an insignificant positive trend of both mean and maximum stomach SUVs with age suggesting that conditions like gastritis commonly found in elderly may contribute to a slightly increased gastric FDG uptake with age.[10] Another study showed the physiologic gastric FDG uptake was significantly higher at the oral end than the aboral end. A stronger gastric FDG uptake at the anal end may therefore be suggestive of a pathologic uptake.[16] One study found that age, fasting period and blood glucose levels did not influence physiologic uptake. However, there seemed to be a patient-specific pattern for stomach and bowel uptake.[17]

In some cases significantly abnormal increase FDG uptake is also noted in patients who have oral positive contrast in the stomach. This artifact is due to over correction of SUV by the presence of oral contrast in attenuated corrected PET images (**Fig. 5**). In such cases one should always look for non-attenuated corrected PET images before calling it abnormal. Other than benign conditions and physiologic FDG uptake, diffuse intense FDG uptake is also noted in patients with lymphoma and linitus plastica. Variable FDG uptake is also noted at pyloric end of stomach (**Fig. 6**). This uptake is seen due to smooth muscle

contraction at pyloric region and is associated with hunger pains.

SMALL BOWEL

The interpretation of abdominal PET images is often difficult due to physiologic uptake of FDG in a variety of abdominal/pelvic organs, which makes it difficult to distinguish normal from abnormal radiotracer uptake. As the intestine remains in a collapsed state, the resolution of the intestine remains very poor on PET-CT (**Fig. 7**). The increased physiologic FDG uptake is primarily due to involuntary smooth muscle motility of intestine (**Fig. 8**). But lymphoid tissue and luminal content due to shed of mucosal cells also contribute to increased FDG uptake in the small intestine. Previously few authors have suggested bowel preparations before PET/PET-CT, but it was not very successful. It has been demonstrated that distension of the intestine is required for better interpretation of images.[18] Combining PET with CT enteroclysis, we evaluated the intestine after its inflation with negative contrast, a technique we call PET-CT enteroclysis. In this pilot study, which included 17 patients with inflammatory bowel disease of the intestine, we assessed the feasibility and diagnostic yield of PET-CT enteroclysis.[19] We found that as a single investigation, PET-CT enteroclysis detects a significantly higher number of lesions both in small and large intestine in comparison to that detected by

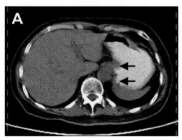 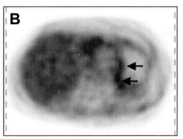 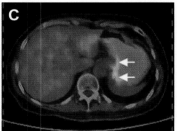

Fig. 4. (A–C) Axial section of CT, PET, and PET-CT images showing mild to moderate FDG uptake in stomach wall (*arrows*).

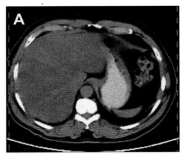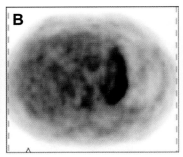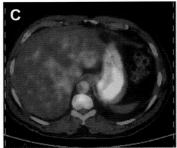

Fig. 5. (*A–C*) Axial CT, PET, and PET-CT images showing intense FDG uptake in stomach wall. This artifact is caused by overcorrection of SUV by the presence of oral contrast in attenuated corrected PET images.

conventional barium studies and colonoscopy combined together. This technique is non-invasive, feasible, very promising. Using PET-CT enteroclysis it is easy to differentiate physiologic FDG uptake from pathologic FDG uptake. In some cases significantly abnormal increase FDG uptake is also noted in patients who have oral positive contrast in the intestine (**Fig. 9**).

Though many a time it is very difficult to differentiate between benign and malignant FDG uptake in the small intestine, following points can be helpful. FDG uptake in inflammatory bowel disease (IBD) is usually diffuse and involve larger segment except stricture where FDG uptake is more focal and involve small segment. Malignant diseases of intestine usually present with mass and obstructive features and involve smaller segment of intestine as compared with those of IBD. The FDG uptake in such patients is focal and more intense.

Studies have found few clinically significant changes in small bowel function with age, in spite of identified statistically significant changes. This possibly reflects the reserve capacity of the organ. Human intestinal permeability has generally been demonstrated to start falling as early as the first week of life and falls throughout childhood.[20,21] Interestingly, infants from a developing nation had intestinal permeability continually increasing

with age, suggesting the influence of environmental factors.[22] Small bowel myenteric neuron density displays an inverse association with age with the largest decrease occurring in the duodenum.[23–25] The propagation velocity of migrating motor complexes also slows, although the amplitude and frequency remain unchanged, with age.[26] Another study suggests an age-associated reduction in contraction frequency after the subjects ingested a meal, while another suggests delayed muscle relaxation in the ilea.[27,28] Small bowel transit times have been variably found to have no correlation or an inverse correlation with age.[29–31]

PET-CT shows a trend toward inverse correlation between age and metabolic activity/FDG uptake, but the trend is not significant. Some or all of the diminution of metabolic activity noted may be secondary to the age-associated decrease in intestinal myenteric neuron density and its possible impact on intestinal muscle function. The study also shows an increase in maximum overall small bowel and colon FDG uptake with age in childhood, which may suggest that such neuronal losses and secondary muscular dysfunction do not begin until adulthood. Indeed, the small bowel and colon of children appear to become more metabolically active with age.[10]

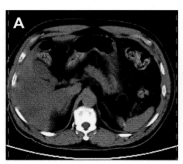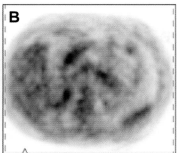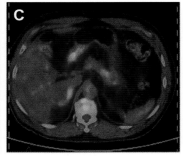

Fig. 6. (*A–C*) Axial section of CT, PET, and PET-CT images showing intense FDG uptake in the pyloric end of stomach.

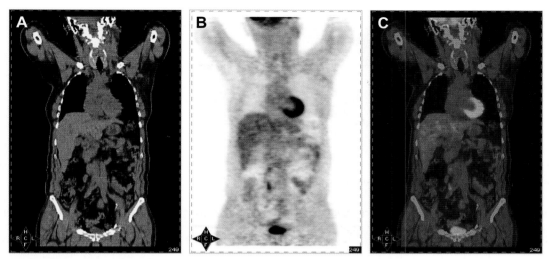

Fig. 7. (A–C) Coronal section of CT, PET, and PET-CT images showing minimal FDG uptake in the intestines. This minimal FDG uptake is caused by smooth muscle contraction of intestines.

COLON AND RECTUM

The physiologic FDG uptake in large bowel is usually more intense than small bowel and commonly involve ascending colon particularly cecum and rectosigmoid colon (**Figs. 10** and **11**). In children pattern of FDG uptake is reversed, FDG uptake is higher in small intestine as compare with large intestine. However, FDG uptake in large intestine is non-specific and unpredictable, many a time the entire colon is visualized especially in the older individuals. Again, to differentiate between benign and malignant FDG uptake in the colon, one should look for pattern of FDG uptake and should take help of CT images of PET-CT studies. FDG uptake in inflammatory bowl disease (IBD) is usually diffuse and involve larger segment except stricture, polyps, diverticulum etc., where FDG uptake is more focal. Colonic cancer usually presents with mass on CT and demonstrate focal area of intense FDG uptake.

The FDG uptake in rectum and anal canal is very commonly seen and is usually higher than physiologic uptake in rest of the small and large intestine (**Figs. 12** and **13**). This increased FDG uptake is due to contraction of smooth muscles of these regions. Many a time inflammatory conditions of rectum and anal canal are also responsible for

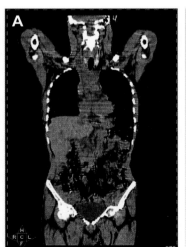
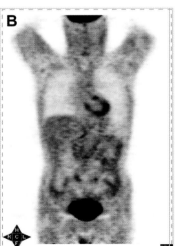
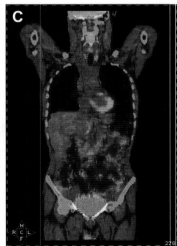

Fig. 8. (A–C) Coronal section of CT, PET, and PET-CT images showing moderate diffuse FDG uptake in the intestines. Note that there is no focal area of intense FDG uptake. Such pattern of FDG uptake in the intestine is a normal variant.

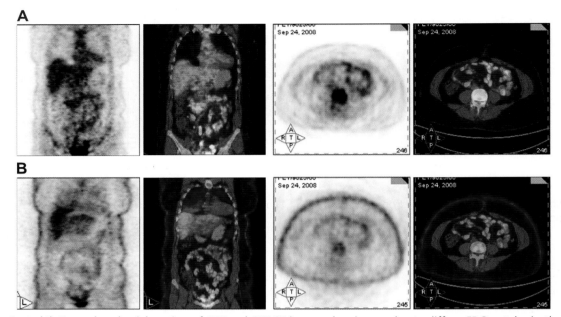

Fig. 9. (A) Coronal and axial section of PET and PET-CT images showing moderate diffuse FDG uptake in the intestines in attenuated corrected images. (B) Minimal FDG uptake is noted in the intestines in the nonattenuated corrected images.

increased FDG uptake eg, polyps, anorectal fistula, fissure etc. Appearance of any mass lesion on CT, which is associated with increased FDG uptake, is often pathologic and needs further evaluation.

Histologically, neuronal density decreases, collagen content increases and structural abnormalities increase in the colonic ganglia with age.[32,33] In the colonic musculature also, collagen content increases and capillary density decreases with age.[34] Slowed colonic transit has been found to affect aging humans.[29,30] The colonic wall as a whole also changes with age, with increasing collagen fibril diameter and overall wall thickness into the third decade.[35,36] Then, with further aging, human colonic wall demonstrates decreasing collagen fibril diameter, particularly in the left colon,

and thus decreasing distal colonic tensile strength.[35,37,38] The collagen fibrils of the left colon also become more tightly packed and cross-linked with age, reducing the elasticity of the walls.[38,39] This diminished elasticity along with a decreased inner colon diameter, contribute to the formation of colonic diverticula in older individuals.[37,39] Perhaps the relative age-associated increase in collagen content within both colonic myenteric ganglia and taenia coli contributes to the decreased metabolic activity in aging distal colon and rectum, as observed in a PET study.[10] The upward trend in ascending colon SUV with age may suggest that either an etiology other than collagen replacement is responsible for altering colonic and rectal metabolic activity there, or that ageing causes collagen deposition preferentially toward the distal

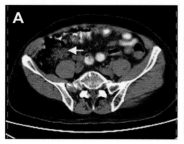
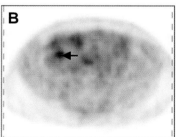
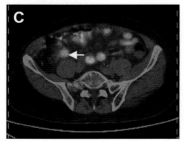

Fig. 10. (A–C) Axial section of CT, PET, and PET-CT images showing intense FDG uptake in the cecum. This is the most common site of physiologic FDG uptake (arrow).

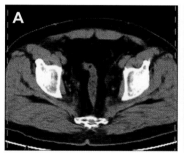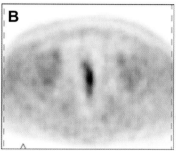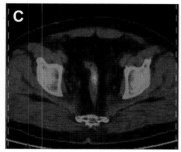

Fig. 11. (A–C) Axial section of CT, PET, and PET-CT images showing intense FDG uptake in the sigmoid colon.

colon and rectum and away from the ascending colon.

LIVER

The FDG uptake noted in attenuated corrected images of liver is usually non-uniform and patchy, which is due to image noise (**Fig. 5**). This non-uniform FDG uptake can mimic or obscure lesions in liver parenchyma. Many inflammatory/infective pathologies can give rise to increased FDG uptake eg, cirrhosis, hepatitis, cholangitis, intrahepatic cholestasis etc. Insulin administration before FDG administration in diabetic patients can also leads to diffuse increased FDG uptake in liver parenchyma. Because of diffuse increased FDG uptake in liver parenchyma and lower FDG uptake in hepatocellular carcinoma, PET/PET-CT has lower sensitivity.

Normally, no FDG uptake is noted in gall bladder. Diffuse uptake in gall bladder wall with out any mass on CT is usually associated with acute or chronic cholecystitis (**Fig. 14**). Focal FDG uptake in gallbladder with mass seen on CT is usually pathologic and associated with gall bladder cancer. However, in few cases this focal FDG uptake can be associated with gall bladder polyp. Biliary tract FDG uptake is usually benign and associated with inflammatory conditions like cholangitis and post stent inflammation.

Conflicting results regarding the relationship between liver volume and subject age have been reported by researchers. A sulfur scintigraphic study of the liver in children showed a linear correlation of liver size with age, weight and both age and weight together. Correlation was found better with weight than with age, with vertical liver dimension showing the best correlation.[40] A study based on Chinese live liver donors used anthropometric data of their body weight and body height for a correlation with liver weights, and found correlation with body weight and gender, with women having smaller livers for the same body weight. Based on this study, a formula for liver weight applicable to

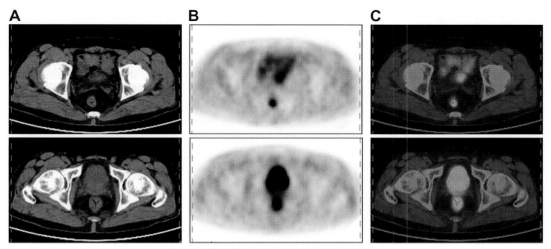

Fig. 12. (A–C) Axial section of CT, PET, and PET-CT images at two different levels showing intense FDG uptake in the rectum. The FDG uptake in rectum and anal canal is very commonly seen and is usually higher than physiologic uptake in the rest of the small and large intestine.

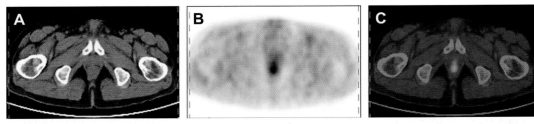

Fig. 13. (*A–C*) Axial section of CT, PET, and PET-CT images showing intense FDG uptake in the anal canal.

the Chinese, based on body weight and gender was derived.[41] Some studies found little or no correlation between liver weight and age.[42] Another study suggested a discrepancy between liver volume estimated by CT and the actual functioning hepatocyte volume in the elderly, which could have serious implications, especially in the post operative scenario.[43] In a study of 149 adults of varying ages (with a median age of nearly 50 years), median volume of the healthy adult liver was found to be 1710.2 mL.[5]

The maximum functional capacity of the liver, as measured by galactose elimination[44] and hepatic

drug clearance,[45] has been found to be reduced in the elderly. This is possibly due to decreased blood flow and a decrease in the intrinsic metabolic activity of the hepatic parenchyma. A decline in liver volume and blood flow and a reduction in vitro and in vivo metabolic capacity have been shown in older subjects, and form the physiologic basis of reduced hepatic drug clearance in this age group.[45] Also noted are an age-associated reduction in bile flow,[46] immunoglobulin secretion into bile[47] and hepatic synthesis of glucose.[48] A PET-CT based study found the hepatic metabolic activity to increase significantly with age in adults,

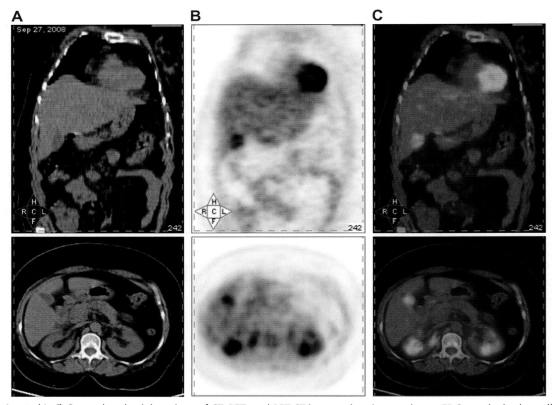

Fig. 14. (*A–C*) Coronal and axial sections of CT, PET, and PET-CT images showing moderate FDG uptake in the gallbladder. Diffuse uptake in gallbladder wall without any mass on CT is usually associated with acute or chronic cholecystitis.

although the overall MVP of the liver did not change significantly.[10] This may reflect an increase in a previously unmeasured aspect of hepatocyte function or inflammatory changes secondary to toxin accumulation. Such generalized inflammatory changes, may also cause the age-associated reduction in liver attenuation noted in the study. No significant relationship was noted between adult liver weight and age.

SPLEEN

Mild diffuse FDG uptake in spleen is physiologic. Similar to liver, FDG uptake in spleen is noted in attenuated corrected images and is usually non-uniform. Normally, FDG uptake in spleen is less than that of liver uptake or same as liver uptake. Rini and colleagues[49] used spleen-to-liver ratio (S/L ratio) for detecting lymphomatous involvement of spleen. A S/L ratio of more than 1.4 was noted in all positive cases, while S/L ratio was 0.8 in both the normal cases. Diffuse increased FDG uptake in spleen is noted in many benign conditions like congestive splenomegaly, giant cell arteritis, post granulocyte colony stimulating factors treatment (G-CSF), post chemotherapy, post blood transfusion, malaria, severe anemia etc. (**Fig. 15**). In patients who receive granulocyte colony stimulating factors treatment, spleen is visualized in more than 50% patients. This diffuse uptake in spleen is less intense as compared with bone marrow uptake. FDG uptake in bone marrow decline much more rapidly than splenic uptake, once G-CSF treatment is stopped. In some case of lymphoma, there can also be diffuse increased FDG uptake in spleen due to lymphoma infiltration. Focal area of increased FDG uptake is commonly associated with malignant pathology, usually lymphoma and metastatic disease. However, on fewer occasion, focal spleen uptake is also noted in patients with splenic abscess and infected hydatid cyst disease.

The relationship between splenic volume and age is also somewhat disputed. A scintigraphic study among pediatric age group has shown correlation of spleen size with child's weight and age, the better correlation being with the weight.[40] Splenic length and multidimensional indexes correlate well with splenic CT volume and also have been used to investigate changes in splenic size with age.[50] An ultrasound based study of a Chinese population showed a rapid growth in splenic length up to the age of 20 years, followed by a mild decrease. It also showed a gender-based variation with the spleens of men being about 0.5 cm longer.[51] Age-associated shortening, thickening, and loss of elastic fibers within the splenic capsule have been suggested to cause the decrease in spleen size with age.[52] Many studies report minimal or insignificant association between splenic size and age.[5,10,42,53] However a CT study revealed that the spleen volume significantly correlated with age, but not with body weight or surface area.[54] Median splenic volume of a population with a median age of nearly 50 years was noted to be 238.3 mL.[5]

Pitted erythrocytes are a marker of splenic dysfunction. One study noted a significantly higher mean percentage of pitted red cells in the elderly over the age of 70 than in the young, suggesting decline in splenic function with age, therefore predisposing to pneumococcal infections.[55] Further

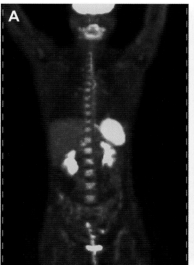
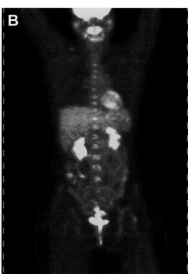

Fig. 15. Projection images of whole-body PET showing intense FDG uptake in the normal-size spleen within 1 week of post–granulocyte colony-stimulating factor treatment (*A*). Follow-up study performed after 12 weeks of completion of chemotherapy shows resolution of splenic FDG uptake (*B*).

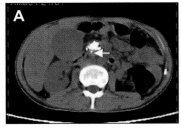
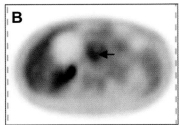
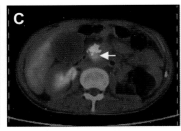

Fig. 16. (*A–C*) Axial section of CT, PET, and PET-CT images showing moderate FDG uptake in the body and head of pancreas in a patient with chronic calcific pancreatitis (*arrow*).

research has shown that splenic function decreases slightly with age but remains clinically intact.[56] Quantitative decrease in a specific splenic cell type has been suggested to cause this decline.[57] In mice, increased apoptotic cell death and decreased proliferative capacity has been suggested in the older spleens.[58] This may contribute to the functional loss in aging spleens, and may also contribute to the age-related decrease in splenic attenuation, observed on CT,[10] due to greater ratio of blood to soft tissue. The reduced flow of blood through the liver may lead to functional congestion of the spleen, further boosting the ratio of blood to soft tissue in the spleen and further decreasing the attenuation of the spleen with age. The same study, however, found no significant change in either splenic FDG uptake or splenic MVP with age. This may reflect that cells within the spleen continue to metabolize glucose despite a waning ability to contribute functionally.

PANCREAS

Minimal diffuse FDG uptake in pancreas is physiologic. Mild to moderate diffuse FDG uptake in pancreas is noted in inflammatory conditions like acute and chronic pancreatitis (**Fig. 16**). Most of the patients of chronic pancreatitis demonstrate calcification on CT as well as decrease in pancreatic volume. Focal FDG uptake in pancreas may be seen in benign and malignant pathologies. We are conducting a study to differentiate benign versus malignant pathologies in pancreatic masses using dual time point imaging with PET-CT. In our experience, benign conditions show rapid wash out of radiotracer when compared with malignant pathology, whereas, malignant conditions of pancreas shows retention or progressive increase in FDG uptake over a period of time.

Studies of age-related changes in pancreas have also reported contradictory findings. An ERCP based study found that aging results in dilation of the accessory pancreatic duct and parts of the main pancreatic duct in individuals over 70 years, although the length of the ducts were similar in all age groups.[59] An endoscopic ultrasound (EUS) study found that the prevalence of EUS abnormalities in patients without clinical evidence of chronic pancreatitis increases with age, particularly after 60 years of age.[60] It suggests possible need to alter the EUS criteria suggestive of pancreatitis. Another study using US showed a positive correlation between age and pancreatic size.[42] However, CT based studies have found no such association.[5] The pancreas of diabetic subjects, especially who are on insulin treatment, have been found to be smaller and more lobulated than those of nondiabetics.[61,62] This size difference is most pronounced in the head and tail regions.[50] No differences in pancreatic attenuation were noted between the two groups.[61] CT of the pancreas might thus help predict which diabetic patients will require insulin therapy A PET-CT study reported no significant correlation of pancreatic size with age. However, it found pancreatic attenuation to be significantly decreased with age.[10] This may be secondary to the fatty replacement of pancreatic tissue, seen in the elderly.

Pancreatic parenchymal perfusion studies using dynamic CT showed a negative correlation with the subject's age, with the perfusion declining over time.[63] However, PET scan fails to show any significant changes in pancreatic FDG uptake, and thus of metabolic function, with age.[10] A fluorescein dilaurate study (a noninvasive test of pancreatic exocrine function) also shows no limitation of pancreatic exocrine function with age.[64] All elderly subjects showed a strictly normal fluorescein dilaurate test, even above 80 years of age.

SUMMARY

Understanding of these normal age-related changes, which can lead to imaging variants and artifacts in structure and function of the human body, is very important. In this article, we reviewed age-associated changes in structural and metabolic function in gastrointestinal tract system, which may be helpful for future clinical or research investigation.

REFERENCES

1. Dang TT, Antolin P, Oxley H. Fiscal implications of ageing: projections of age-related spending. Economics Department Working Papers No. 305. Organization for Economic Cooperation and Development, 2001.
2. Tietz NW, Shuey DF, Wekstein DR. Laboratory values in fit aging individuals: sexagenarians through centenarians. Clin Chem 1992;38:1167–85.
3. Heymsfield SB, Fulenwider T, Nordlinger B, et al. Accurate measurement of liver, kidney, and spleen volume and mass by computerized axial tomography. Ann Intern Med 1979;90:185–7.
4. Urata K, Kawasaki S, Matsunami H, et al. Calculation of child and adult standard liver volume for liver transplantation. Hepatology 1995;21:1317–21.
5. Geraghty EM, Boone JM, McGahan JP, et al. Normal organ volume assessment from abdominal CT. Abdom Imaging 2004;29:482–90.
6. Jackowski C, Thali MJ, Buck U, et al. Noninvasive estimation of organ weights by postmortem magnetic resonance imaging and multislice computed tomography. Invest Radiol 2006;41:572–8.
7. Kumar R, Nadig M, Chauhan A. Positron emission tomography: clinical application in oncology: part I. Expert Rev Anticancer Ther 2005;5:1079–94.
8. Kumar R, Dadparvar S. FDG-PET/PET-CT in carcinoma of cervix. Cancer 2007;110(8):1650–3.
9. Kumar R, Xiu Y, Potenta S, et al. FDG-PET in evaluation of treatment response in patients with gastrointestinal tract lymphomas. J Nucl Med 2004;45(11):1796–803.
10. Meier JM, Alavi A, Iruvuri S, et al. Assessment of age-related changes in abdominal organ structure and function with computed tomography and positron emission tomography. Semin Nucl Med 2007;37:154–72.
11. Fulp SR, Dalton CB, Castell JA, et al. Aging-related alterations in human upper esophageal sphincter function. Am J Gastroenterol 1990;85:1569–72.
12. Grande L, Lacima G, Ros E, et al. Deterioration of esophageal motility with age: a manometric study of 79 healthy subjects. Am J Gastroenterol 1999;94:1795–801.
13. Ren J, Shaker R, Kusano M, et al. Effect of aging on the secondary esophageal peristalsis: presbyesophagus revisited. Am J Physiol 1995;268:G772–9.
14. Hollis JB, Castell DO. Esophageal function in elderly man: a new look at presbyesophagus. Ann Intern Med 1974;80:371–4.
15. Salaun PY, Grewal RK, Dodamane I, et al. An analysis of the 18F-FDG uptake pattern in the stomach. J Nucl Med 2005;46:48–51.
16. Koga H, Sasaki M, Kuwabara Y, et al. An analysis of the physiological FDG uptake pattern in the stomach. Ann Nucl Med 2003;17:733–8.
17. de Groot M, Meeuwis AP, Kok PJ, et al. Influence of blood glucose level, age and fasting period on non-pathological FDG uptake in heart and gut. Eur J Nucl Med Mol Imaging 2005;32:98–101.
18. Prabhakar HB, Sahani DV, Fischman AJ, et al. Bowel hot spots at PET-CT. Radiographics 2007;27:145–59.
19. Das CJ, Makharia G, Kumar R, et al. PET-CT-enteroclysis: a new technique for evaluation of inflammatory diseases of the intestine. Eur J Nucl Med Mol Imaging 2007;34:2106–14.
20. Catassi C, Bonucci A, Coppa GV, et al. Intestinal permeability changes during the first month: effect of natural versus artificial feeding. J Pediatr Gastroenterol Nutr 1995;21:383–6.
21. Kalach N, Rocchiccioli F, de Boissieu D, et al. Intestinal permeability in children: variation with age and reliability in the diagnosis of cow's milk allergy. Acta Paediatr 2001;90:499–504.
22. Goto K, Chew F, Torun B, et al. Epidemiology of altered intestinal permeability to lactulose and mannitol in Guatemalan infants. J Pediatr Gastroenterol Nutr 1999;28:282–90.
23. Phillips RJ, Powley TL. As the gut ages: timetables for aging of innervation vary by organ in the Fischer 344 rat. J Comp Neurol 2001;434:358–77.
24. Wester T, O'Briain DS, Puri P. Notable postnatal alterations in the myenteric plexus of normal human bowel. Gut 1999;44:666–74.
25. de Souza RR, Moratelli HB, Borges N, et al. Age-induced nerve cell loss in the myenteric plexus of the small intestine in man. Gerontology 1993;39:183–8.
26. Husebye E, Engedal K. The patterns of motility are maintained in the human small intestine throughout the process of aging. Scand J Gastroenterol 1992;27:397–404.
27. Anuras S, Sutherland J. Small intestinal manometry in healthy elderly subjects. J Am Geriatr Soc 1984;32:581–3.
28. Smits GJ, Lefebvre RA. Influence of age on cholinergic and inhibitory nonadrenergic noncholinergic responses in the rat ileum. Eur J Pharmacol 1996;303:79–86.
29. Madsen JL. Effects of gender, age, and body mass index on gastrointestinal transit times. Dig Dis Sci 1992;37:1548–53.
30. Graff J, Brinch K, Madsen JL. Gastrointestinal mean transit times in young and middle-aged healthy subjects. Clin Physiol 2001;21:253–9.
31. Smits GJ, Lefebvre RA. Influence of aging on gastric emptying of liquids, small intestine transit, and fecal output in rats. Exp Gerontol 1996;31:589–96.
32. Gomes OA, de Souza RR, Liberti EA. A preliminary investigation of the effects of aging on the nerve cell number in the myenteric ganglia of the human colon. Gerontology 1997;43:210–7.

33. Hanani M, Fellig Y, Udassin R, et al. Age-related changes in the morphology of the myenteric plexus of the human colon. Auton Neurosci 2004;113:71–8.

34. Gabella G. Development and ageing of intestinal musculature and nerves: the guinea-pig taenia coli. J Neurocytol 2001;30:733–66.

35. Parry DA, Barnes GR, Craig AS. A comparison of the size distribution of collagen fibrils in connective tissues as a function of age and a possible relation between fibril size distribution and mechanical properties. Proc R Soc Lond B Biol Sci 1978;203:305–21.

36. Haber HP, Stern M. Intestinal ultrasonography in children and young adults: bowel wall thickness is age dependent. J Ultrasound Med 2000;19:315–21.

37. Watters DA, Smith AN, Eastwood MA, et al. Mechanical properties of the colon: comparison of the features of the African and European colon in vitro. Gut 1985;26:384–92.

38. Thomson HJ, Busuttil A, Eastwood MA, et al. Submucosal collagen changes in the normal colon and in diverticular disease. Int J Colorectal Dis 1987;2:208–13.

39. Wess L, Eastwood MA, Wess TJ, et al. Cross linking of collagen is increased in colonic diverticulosis. Gut 1995;37:91–4.

40. Markisz JA, Treves ST, Davis RT. Normal hepatic and splenic size in children: scintigraphic determination. Pediatr Radiol 1987;17:273–6.

41. Chan SC, Liu CL, Lo CM, et al. Estimating liver weight of adults by body weight and gender. World J Gastroenterol 2006;12:2217–22.

42. Niederau C, Sonnenberg A, Muller JE, et al. Sonographic measurements of the normal liver, spleen, pancreas, and portal vein. Radiology 1983;149:537–40.

43. Wakabayashi H, Nishiyama Y, Ushiyama T, et al. Evaluation of the effect of age on functioning hepatocyte mass and liver blood flow using liver scintigraphy in preoperative estimations for surgical patients: comparison with CT volumetry. J Surg Res 2002;106:246–53.

44. Marchesini G, Bua V, Brunori A, et al. Galactose elimination capacity and liver volume in aging man. Hepatology 1988;8:1079–83.

45. Zeeh J, Platt D. The aging liver: structural and functional changes and their consequences for drug treatment in old age. Gerontology 2002;48:121–7.

46. Handler JA, Genell CA, Goldstein RS. Hepatobiliary function in senescent male Sprague-Dawley rats. Hepatology 1994;19:1496–503.

47. Schmucker DL, Gilbert R, Jones AL, et al. Effect of aging on the hepatobiliary transport of dimeric immunoglobulin A in the male Fischer rat. Gastroenterology 1985;88:436–43.

48. Sastre J, Pallardo FV, Pla R, et al. Aging of the liver: age-associated mitochondrial damage in intact hepatocytes. Hepatology 1996;24:1199–205.

49. Rini JN, Leonidas JC, Tomas MB, et al. 18F-FDG PET versus CT for evaluating the spleen during initial staging of lymphoma. J Nucl Med 2003;44(7):1072–4.

50. Bezerra AS, D'Ippolito G, Faintuch S, et al. Determination of splenomegaly by CT: is there a place for a single measurement? AJR Am J Roentgenol 2005;184:1510–3.

51. Loftus WK, Metreweli C. Normal splenic size in a Chinese population. J Ultrasound Med 1997;16:345–7.

52. Rodrigues CJ, Sacchetti JC, Rodrigues AJ Jr. Age-related changes in the elastic fiber network of the human splenic capsule. Lymphology 1999;32:64–9.

53. Prassopoulos P, Daskalogiannaki M, Raissaki M, et al. Determination of normal splenic volume on computed tomography in relation to age, gender and body habitus. Eur Radiol 1997;7:246–8.

54. Kaneko J, Sugawara Y, Matsui Y, et al. Normal splenic volume in adults by computed tomography. Hepatogastroenterology 2002;49:1726–7.

55. Markus HS, Toghill PJ. Impaired splenic function in elderly people. Age Ageing 1991;20:287–90.

56. Ravaglia G, Forti P, Biagi F, et al. Splenic function in old age. Gerontology 1998;44:91–4.

57. Chinnaiyan AM, O'Rourke K, Yu GL, et al. Signal transduction by DR3, a death domain-containing receptor related to TNFR-1 and CD95. Science 1996;274:990–2.

58. Itzhaki O, Skutelsky E, Kaptzan T, et al. Ageing-apoptosis relation in murine spleen. Mech Ageing Dev 2003;124:999–1012.

59. Anand BS, Vij JC, Mac HS, et al. Effect of aging on the pancreatic ducts: a study based on endoscopic retrograde pancreatography. Gastrointest Endosc 1989;35:210–3.

60. Rajan E, Clain JE, Levy MJ, et al. Age-related changes in the pancreas identified by EUS: a prospective evaluation. Gastrointest Endosc 2005;61:401–6.

61. Gilbeau JP, Poncelet V, Libon E, et al. The density, contour, and thickness of the pancreas in diabetics: CT findings in 57 patients. AJR Am J Roentgenol 1992;159:527–31.

62. Migdalis IN, Voudouris G, Kalogeropoulou K, et al. Size of the pancreas in non-insulin-dependent diabetic patients. J Med 1991;22:179–86.

63. Tsushima Y, Kusano S. Age-dependent decline in parenchymal perfusion in the normal human pancreas: measurement by dynamic computed tomography. Pancreas 1998;17:148–52.

64. Gullo L, Ventrucci M, Naldoni P, et al. Aging and exocrine pancreatic function. J Am Geriatr Soc 1986;34:790–2.

PET and PET/CT in the Diagnosis and Staging of Esophageal and Gastric Cancers

Jeremy J. Erasmus, MBBCh[a,b,]*, Eric M. Rohren, MD, PhD[b,c], Roland Hustinx, MD, PhD[d]

KEYWORDS

• Esophageal cancer • Gastric cancer • FDG • PET-CT

The incidence of cancers of the distal esophagus and the gastric cardia is increasing in developed countries, and esophageal and gastric cancers are among the leading causes of cancer-related deaths worldwide.[1] Radical surgical resection is the primary curative treatment for early esophageal and gastric cancers; however, there are numerous treatment options. Multimodality treatment that employs preoperative chemotherapy with or without radiation followed by surgical resection in suitable candidates is increasingly being used in patients who have locally advanced cancer.[2–5] This evolving treatment strategy, together with the substantial morbidity and mortality associated with surgical resection, makes appropriate patient selection important for optimal management. In fact, management is determined to a large extent by patient performance status, location of the primary cancer, and stage of disease at presentation. Accordingly, accurate determination of the anatomic extent of the primary tumor and nodal and distant metastases is important.

Patients who have esophageal and gastric cancers are usually staged before therapy according to the recommendations of the American Joint Commission on Cancer (AJCC)/Union Internationale Contre le Cancer (UICC) system for pathologic and clinical staging, which follows a standardized evaluation of the primary tumor (T), regional lymph nodes (N), and distant metastatic disease (M). The clinical staging of esophageal and gastric cancers is usually performed using endoscopy or endoscopic ultrasound (EUS) and CT.[6–15] PET with fludeoxyglucose F 18 (FDG) is being increasingly used in the initial staging of patients who have esophageal and gastric cancers and may have a role in the assessment of therapeutic response. Because of the poor spatial resolution of PET compared with CT, however, the accurate assessment of the primary tumor and localization of nodal metastases and the detection of small pulmonary metastases are often difficult. Integrated PET-CT imaging with coregistration of anatomic and functional imaging data can improve the localization of regions of increased FDG uptake and the accuracy of staging in patients who have esophageal cancer.[16,17] MR imaging is infrequently used in the imaging algorithm of esophageal and gastric cancers; however, advances in MR imaging, including the use of high-resolution T2-weighted techniques and the recent development of endoluminal imaging, may result in MR imaging becoming useful in the staging of the primary esophageal cancer.[18–20] This

[a] Department of Diagnostic Radiology, Unit 57, The University of Texas M.D. Anderson Cancer Center, 1515 Holcombe Boulevard, Houston, TX 77030, USA
[b] Division of Diagnostic Imaging, Unit 0371, The University of Texas M.D. Anderson Cancer Center, 1515 Holcombe Boulevard, Houston, TX 77030, USA
[c] Department of Nuclear Medicine, The University of Texas M.D. Anderson Cancer Center, 1515 Holcombe Boulevard, Houston, TX 77030, USA
[d] Service de Médecine Nucléaire, Centre Hospitalier Universitaire, Sart Tilman B35, 4000 Liège, Belgium
* Corresponding author. Division of Diagnostic Imaging, Unit 0371, The University of Texas M.D. Anderson Cancer Center, 1515 Holcombe Boulevard, Houston, TX 77030.
E-mail address: jerasmus@di.mdacc.tmc.edu (J.J. Erasmus).

PET Clin 3 (2008) 135–145
doi:10.1016/j.cpet.2008.09.002

article reviews the appropriate role of FDG-PET and FDG-PET-CT imaging in the diagnosis, initial staging, and detection of recurrent disease in patients who have esophageal and gastric cancers.

ESOPHAGEAL CANCER

The findings of two recent meta-analyses reviewing the staging investigations for esophageal cancer provide an indication of the overall roles that EUS, CT, and FDG-PET have in the evaluation of patients who have esophageal cancer.[8,13] EUS with fine-needle aspiration biopsy is the optimal modality for the detection and evaluation of the primary tumor and the detection of regional lymph node metastases (sensitivities for EUS, CT, and FDG-PET are 80%, 50%, and 57%, respectively; specificities are 70%, 83%, and 85%, respectively). FDG-PET and CT are useful in the detection of distant metastases (sensitivities are 71% and 52%, respectively; specificities are 93% and 91%, respectively). The following sections expand and clarify aspects of the findings of these meta-analyses as they pertain to the imaging performed in the clinical staging of patients who have esophageal cancer.

Diagnosis

Primary tumor detection by FDG-PET imaging has historically been considered high (greater than 90%) in patients who have esophageal carcinoma; however, the limitations in the spatial resolution of PET imaging and the stage and size of the primary tumor at presentation affect the accuracy of detection.[21–23] In a recent study by Kato and colleagues[22] comparing FDG-PET imaging with CT for staging patients who have esophageal cancer, the uptake of FDG was related to the stage of the primary esophageal tumor. Overall, FDG uptake in the primary tumor was visualized in 119 of 149 patients (80%) at initial evaluation. In the 81 patients who were treated with curative resection, FDG uptake was detected in 17 of 40 (43%) T1 tumors, 83% of T2 tumors, 97% of T3 tumors, and 100% of T4 tumors (**Figs. 1** and **2**). Himeno and colleagues[21] reported that FGD-PET imaging could reliably detect the primary esophageal tumor when the stage was T1b (invasion of the submucosa) or higher but could not detect tumors with less locoregional invasion (ie, Tis [in situ] and T1a tumors [invasion of the muscularis mucosae]).

The limitations of esophageal tumor detection by PET imaging are greater in the assessment of superficial esophageal cancers because these tumors are typically small. In this regard, in a recent study, Little and colleagues[23] reported that FDG-PET imaging had a poor detection rate for superficial esophageal cancers. In 58 patients who had superficial tumors, only 31 (53%) had increased FDG uptake in the primary esophageal tumor (median standardized uptake value 3.5, range 2.1–16.6). Similarly, Miyata and colleagues[24] reported that only 21 of 41 patients

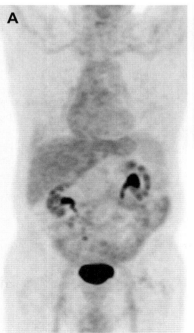

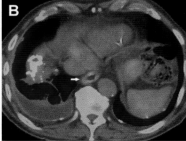

Fig. 1. Early-stage esophageal cancer (T1a—invasion of the muscularis mucosae) in an 83-year-old man in which the primary esophageal tumor is not visualized on PET-CT imaging. (A) Whole-body maximum-intensity projection image shows FDG uptake in the esophagus and absence of nodal and distant metastases. (B) Axial integrated PET-CT shows a normal-appearing esophagus with background uptake of FDG in the region of the primary esophageal cancer (arrow). Note that right pleural effusion and pleural calcification are a manifestation of asbestos exposure.

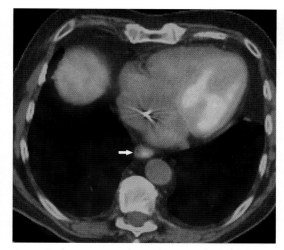

Fig. 2. Early-stage esophageal cancer (T1b—invasion of the submucosa) in an 81-year-old man in which the primary esophageal tumor has increased uptake of FDG on PET imaging. Axial integrated PET-CT shows focal increased uptake of FDG (maximum standardized uptake value 5.8) by the primary esophageal cancer. Note that FDG-PET imaging has a poor detection rate for T1 esophageal tumors.

(51.2%) who had superficial esophageal cancers had increased FDG uptake in the primary esophageal tumor.

Initial Staging

Patients who have esophageal cancer are typically staged before therapy according to the recommendations of the AJCC and UICC 2002 guidelines for pathologic and clinical staging (**Box 1**).[25] Because of the limitations of CT and PET imaging in the assessment of the primary tumor (T), it is the comprehensive understanding of the descriptors used for lymph node involvement (N) and metastatic disease (M) that is important in the appropriate use and interpretation of PET and PET-CT imaging. In this regard, the N1 descriptor for regional nodes includes paraesophageal and abdominal nodes cephalad to the celiac axis, with the important understanding that these nodal metastases do not preclude surgical resection. M1 disease is subdivided into nonregional lymph nodes (M1a) and distant metastases (M1b). An exception to subdividing M1 disease is when the primary cancer is located in the midesophagus, because nodal metastases in this subset of patients have a similar prognosis as hematogenous metastases to other distant sites (see **Box 1**). It is important to note that the designation of distant metastatic disease (M1b) from nonregional nodal

---

Box 1
American Joint Committee on Cancer TNM staging system for esophageal cancer

T—Primary tumor
  TX Primary tumor cannot be assessed

  T0 No evidence of primary tumor

  Tis Carcinoma in situ

  T1 Tumor invades lamina propria or submucosa

  T2 Tumor invades muscularis propria

  T3 Tumor invades adventitia

  T4 Tumor invades adjacent structures

N—Regional lymph nodes
  NX Regional lymph nodes cannot be assessed

  N0 No regional lymph node metastasis

  N1 Regional lymph node metastasis

M—Distant metastasis
  MX Distant metastasis cannot be assessed

  M0 No distant metastasis

M1 Distant metastasis

  Tumors of the lower thoracic esophagus

   M1a Metastasis in celiac lymph nodes

   M1b Other distant metastasis

  Tumors of the midthoracic esophagus

   M1a Not applicable[a]

   M1b Nonregional lymph nodes and other distant metastasis

  Tumors of the upper thoracic esophagus:

   M1a Metastasis in cervical nodes

   M1b Other distant metastasis

[a] For tumors of midthoracic esophagus, only M1b is used because these tumors with metastasis in nonregional lymph nodes have an equally poor prognosis as those with metastasis in other distant sites.
Adapted from American Joint Committee on Cancer: AJCC Cancer Staging Manual. 6th ed. New York, NY: Springer, 2002, pp 91–98; with permission.

---

disease (M1a) also depends on the location of the primary esophageal tumor (**Fig. 3**; see **Box 1**).

Small studies have reported a 3% to 22% change in management due to the addition of FDG-PET imaging to the preoperative assessment of patients who have esophageal cancer.[26–32] FDG-PET imaging followed by EUS has been proposed as the most cost-effective strategy in the preoperative staging and management of patients who have esophageal cancer.[12,33] The precise role of FDG-PET and PET-CT in the staging

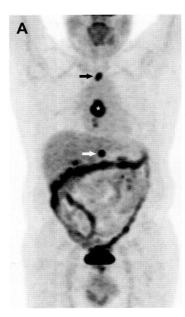

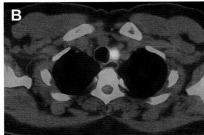

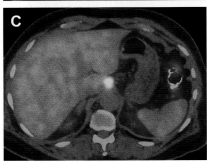

Fig. 3. Distant metastases in a 67-year-old man who had a midesophageal cancer. (*A*) Whole-body maximum-intensity projection image shows increased FDG uptake in the primary esophageal cancer (*asterisk*) and nonregional lymph nodes (*arrows*). (*B, C*) Axial integrated PET-CT shows increased uptake of FDG in metastases in a superior mediastinal node and a left gastric node. Note that metastases in nonregional lymph nodes are considered distant metastases (M1b) when the tumor is located in the midesophagus.

algorithm of patients who have potentially resectable esophageal cancer is not clearly defined, however. In the authors' experience, the optimal imaging/staging strategy is a combination of EUS, contrast-enhanced CT of the chest and abdomen, and integrated PET-CT imaging. The following sections review the use of PET and PET-CT imaging in the clinical staging of patients who have esophageal cancer.

Primary Tumor

The extent of the primary tumor is categorized as T1 through T4 according to the depth of tumor penetration into the esophageal wall (see **Box 1**). The assessment of local tumor invasion is one of the most significant factors in determining appropriate treatment. PET and PET-CT offer little information regarding the depth of invasion, due to the spatial resolution limits of the scan. Furthermore, there is no consistent relationship between the intensity of FDG uptake and the depth of tumor invasion (T staging). Although FDG uptake and T staging are positively related, this association is poor.[21–23,28,34,35] This poor association is largely due to the fact that the intensity of FDG uptake is determined by the metabolic activity of the tumor and the volume of the tumor mass, whereas T staging is a based on a unidimensional measurement of the depth of invasion of the tumor. The inability to differentiate between T1, T2, and T3 parameters and the poor ability to identify invasion of adjacent structures that would preclude resection (T4 disease) are major limitations in the use of PET and PET-CT in evaluation of the primary tumor. In this regard, Lowe and colleagues[14] reported that local tumor staging (T) was done correctly by CT and PET in only 42% of patients who had esophageal cancer (compared with 71% who underwent EUS). Furthermore, in a study by Little and colleagues[23] that evaluated 58 patients who had superficial esophageal cancers to determine whether FDG-PET-CT imaging could accurately classify the primary tumor (T), including distinguishing high-grade dysplasia (Tis) from invasive cancer (T1), PET could not differentiate Tis from T1. Of interest, increased FDG uptake was detected more frequently with increasing depth of tumor invasion (5/11 [45%] for Tis compared with 11/16 [69%] for T1), and the standardized uptake value also increased (median 0 for Tis compared with 2.7 for T1) (see **Figs. 1** and **2**). The results of this study led the investigators to conclude that not only should PET not be used in the T staging of patients who have superficial esophageal tumors but FDG-PET imaging is also not indicated in the overall T, N, and M staging of superficial esophageal tumors because of the poor sensitivity in detecting nodal metastases and the low prevalence of distant metastases in these patients.

In the evaluation of the primary esophageal tumor, FDG-PET may also have a potential role in the determination of the length of the tumor.[36] The accurate delineation of the superior and inferior extent of viable esophageal tumor is important in radiotherapy planning, and tumor length is also a strong independent predictor of prognosis in patients who have esophageal cancer.[37–40]

Griffiths and colleagues[38] reported that a tumor length greater than 3.5 cm is associated with a worse stage of disease at presentation and with poor overall survival. Currently, tumor length is measured by EUS; however, accurate clinical delineation of tumor length can be difficult. Mamede and colleagues[36] recently evaluated a three-dimensional tumor segmentation method using FDG-PET to estimate metabolic esophageal tumor length and its correlation with the length observed in surgical specimens. Their preliminary report in 17 patients who underwent primary esophageal resection showed that FDG-PET–derived tumor metabolic lengths correlated well with tumor length assessed by EUS and surgical pathology results.

Regional Lymph Nodes

Nodal metastases in a paraesophageal location adjacent to the primary tumor are considered regional nodal metastases (N1). Abdominal nodes cephalad to the celiac axis are also designated N1 when the primary esophageal cancer is located in the distal esophagus, and these nodes do not preclude surgical resection (see **Box 1**). EUS with or without transesophageal endoscopic biopsy of nodes is routinely performed to determine the presence of locoregional nodal metastases.[8,11–15] CT has poor sensitivity and specificity in the detection of N1 disease, and the addition of FDG-PET to the imaging algorithm of patients who have esophageal cancer has not significantly improved N1 nodal staging.[14,15,41] The sensitivity of PET in the detection of nodal metastatic disease is overall poor (**Fig. 4**).[14,22,28,42,43] In a recent meta-analysis of 12 studies concerning the value of FDG-PET in the preoperative staging of patients who have esophageal cancer, the pooled sensitivity and specificity values for the detection of locoregional nodal disease were 51% and 84%, respectively.[26] In addition, in a recent prospective study to assess preoperative staging in patients who had esophageal cancer, Flamen and colleagues[28] compared the accuracy FDG-PET with conventional noninvasive modalities. In 39 of 74 patients who underwent a two- or three-field lymphadenectomy in conjunction with primary curative esophagectomy, FDG-PET sensitivity, specificity, and accuracy in the detection of regional nodal metastasis were 33%, 89%, and 59%, respectively. It is important to note that FDG-PET did not lead to an increase in accuracy of regional nodal staging compared with the current standard of combined CT and EUS.

Metastatic Disease

Distant metastases are common in patients with esophageal cancer who are being considered for

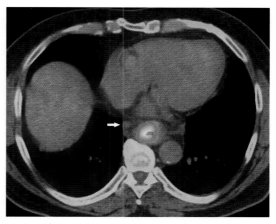

Fig. 4. False-negative PET-CT in regional nodal metastasis in a 55-year-old man who had distal esophageal cancer. Axial integrated PET-CT shows increased uptake of FDG in the primary esophageal cancer. Note the 1-cm regional lymph nodes with background FDG activity (*arrow*). EUS-guided biopsy revealed nodal metastatic disease. Note that the sensitivity of PET in the detection of nodal metastatic disease is not optimal and does not improve the accuracy of regional nodal staging compared with the combined use of CT and EUS.

surgical resection. Accurate determination of the M stage is important because these patients do not benefit from surgical resection. EUS and CT imaging of the chest and abdomen are typically performed to detect these metastases.[12,14,26,44–46] FDG-PET imaging may be more accurate than conventional imaging with CT and EUS in the detection of distant metastatic disease at presentation in patients who have esophageal cancer. Flamen and colleagues[28] reported that FDG-PET had a superior accuracy (82%) for the diagnosis of distant lymph node involvement or organ metastasis compared with the combined use of CT and EUS (64%). In a study by Lowe and colleagues,[14] the sensitivity and specificity for distant metastases were reported to be 81% and 82% for CT, 73% and 86% for EUS, and 81% and 91% for PET. Recent studies suggest that the addition of PET imaging to the staging algorithm improves the accuracy of preoperative staging and prevents inappropriate esophageal resection (**Figs. 5** and **6**).[15,27,28,33,47–51] In this regard, PET imaging has been reported to detect distant nodal and organ metastases in up to 20% of patients who are initially considered to have resectable disease based on conventional staging.[27]

A prospective multi-institutional trial study by the American College of Surgeons Oncology Group, however, has reported little additional value of including FDG-PET imaging in the staging

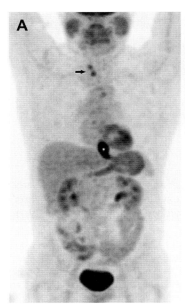

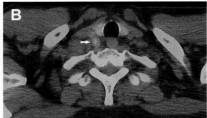

Fig. 5. Nonregional nodal metastases in a 57-year-old man who had distal esophageal cancer. (A) Whole-body maximum-intensity projection image shows increased FDG uptake in the primary esophageal cancer (*asterisk*) and nonregional lymph nodes (*arrow*). (B) Axial integrated PET-CT shows increased uptake of FDG in metastases in a right supraclavicular node (*arrow*) and a superior mediastinal node (not shown). Note that metastases in nonregional lymph nodes are considered distant metastases (M1a).

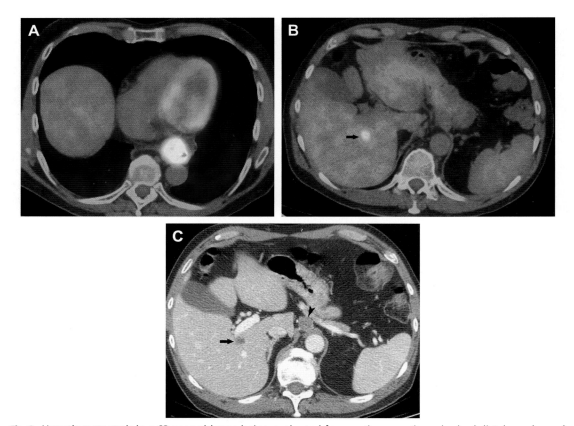

Fig. 6. Hepatic metastasis in a 63-year-old man being evaluated for curative resection who had distal esophageal cancer. (A, B) Axial integrated PET-CT shows increased uptake of FDG in the distal esophageal cancer and focal increased FDG-uptake in a hepatic metastasis (M1b) (*arrow*). (C) Contrast-enhanced CT of the abdomen shows a small, low-attenuation lesion in the liver (*arrow*) that is suspicious, but not diagnostic, for a metastasis. Note the enlarged left gastric node due to N1 metastatic disease (*arrowhead*). Integrated PET-CT improves the accuracy of staging because of the ability to detect distant metastases.

of patients who have resectable esophageal cancer after completion of routine staging procedures.[48] PET imaging identified biopsy-proven unsuspected distant metastatic disease in only 4.8% of the patients after complete conventional staging was performed. An additional 3.7% of the patients, however, had unconfirmed PET-detected distant metastases (M1b disease) and were treated nonsurgically. Overall, there were 9.5% of patients who had apparent PET-detected metastases in which histologic confirmation was not obtained. Accordingly, the overall rate of detected metastases could be as high as 14.3%; however, it is unlikely that all the patients who had unconfirmed metastatic disease had metastases, because many of these patients subsequently underwent successful surgical resection. At least 3.7% of patients who had findings of distant metastases on PET imaging were falsely positive, and accordingly, PET findings suspicious for metastases should be confirmed before excluding a patient from surgical consideration. It is of interest that the impact of PET on surgical resection in this study extended further than the detection of M1 disease: several patients did not undergo resection after PET revealed multistation nodal metastases (N1).

In a more recent prospective study by van Westreenen and colleagues,[52] FDG-PET imaging performed after a preoperative staging protocol that included multidetector CT, EUS, and sonography of the neck revealed distant metastases in only 8 of 199 (4%) of the patients who had esophageal cancer and prevented unnecessary resection in only 3% because all these patients had advanced disease. There was also a high rate of false-positive PET findings (7.5%) that resulted in unnecessary additional investigations. Accordingly, the investigators concluded that although FDG-PET improves the selection of patients who have esophageal cancer for curative resection, the diagnostic benefit is limited after comprehensive conventional staging.

Diagnosis of Recurrent Esophageal Cancer

Recurrence of esophageal cancer is common after curative surgical resection and typically occurs within 2 years after resection.[53] Although locoregional recurrence of malignancy is not uncommon, most patients present with distant metastases.[28,54,55] Because the survival of patients who have recurrent esophageal cancer is poor and the treatment options are limited, routine surveillance imaging for recurrent malignancy is not usually performed in asymptomatic patients; however, early detection of recurrent disease may be beneficial because treatment may prolong tumor-free survival.[56]

Flamen and colleagues[28] reported preliminary work indicating that FDG-PET imaging has a high sensitivity for detecting recurrent malignancy after curative resection of cancer of the esophagus or gastroesophageal junction. In their study, perianastomotic, regional, and distant recurrent esophageal cancer was found in 33 of 41 patients who had clinical or radiologic findings suspicious for recurrent disease. FDG-PET has an overall sensitivity of 95% for the detection of locoregional and distant metastases; however, PET did not improve the diagnostic accuracy for locoregional recurrences compared with conventional imaging. FDG-PET imaging was inaccurate for the diagnosis of perianastomotic recurrence due to frequent false-positive FDG uptake as a result of inflammation (sensitivity 100%, specificity 57%, and accuracy 74% compared with 100%, 93%, and 96%, respectively, for conventional diagnostic work-up) (**Fig. 7**). For the diagnosis of regional and distant recurrences, the sensitivity, specificity, and accuracy of PET were 94%, 82%, and 87%, respectively, compared with 81%, 82%, and 81%, respectively, for conventional diagnostic work-up. Overall, PET provided additional information in 11 of 41 (27%) patients and had a major impact on diagnosis in 5 patients by confirming malignancy that was equivocal or negative on diagnostic work-up (**Fig. 8**).

PET-CT imaging can also detect distant metastases after neoadjuvant therapy and before planned esophagectomy. A few small studies have reported that detection of metastases occurs in up to 17% of these patients.[57–59] In a more recent study, Bruzzi and colleagues[60,61] reported that PET-CT imaging detected metastatic disease in 7 of 88 patients (8%) who had potentially resectable esophageal carcinoma after neoadjuvant therapy. Of clinical relevance, in 2 of 7 patients, the use of PET imaging allowed detection of metastases that were not detected on conventional staging. In addition, similar to a previous report by these investigators, metastatic disease also occurred in an unusual site (skeletal muscle). The investigators concluded that because the metastases can be clinically occult and in unusual and uncommon locations after induction therapy, whole-body PET-CT is the best imaging method for their detection.

GASTRIC CANCER

Although gastric cancer is among the most common malignant diseases worldwide, it is much less frequent in the United States and Europe.[1]

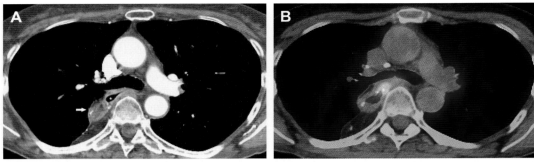

Fig. 7. False-positive FDG uptake in perianastomotic inflammation in a 74-year-old woman after resection of esophageal cancer. (*A*) Contrast-enhanced CT shows normal appearance of the anastomosis of the residual native esophagus (*asterisk*) and gastric conduit (*arrow*) 11 months after esophagectomy. (*B*) Axial integrated PET-CT shows focal increased uptake of FDG uptake in the region of the anastomosis that is suspicious for local recurrence of malignancy. Endoscopic biopsy revealed acute and chronic inflammation and no malignancy. Note that FDG-PET imaging is inaccurate for the diagnosis of perianastomotic recurrence due to frequent false-positive FDG-uptake as a result of inflammation.

Gastric cancer is often diagnosed at an advanced stage, with most resected gastric carcinomas having already spread to the regional lymph nodes. For staging purposes, the classification system used in the Western world is the AJCC/UICC system, which relies on the local invasion (T), number of lymph node metastases (N), and presence of distant metastases (M).

FDG-PET performs poorly for diagnosing gastric cancer, with a sensitivity ranging from 60% to 91%.[62,63] The intensity of uptake is variable and tends to be lower in mucinous carcinomas and signet ring cell carcinomas than in other pathologic types.[62] Compared with other techniques such as endoscopy, EUS, and CT, PET has no role for evaluating the T stage of the disease. Few data are available regarding PET for nodal staging, but the sensitivity appears to be extremely low.[64,65] On the other hand, PET is more specific than CT, especially for assessing the proximal lymph node status, and it may change the clinical management by detecting additional distal lesions in patients initially selected for surgery.[66,67] The added value of PET-CT over PET has not yet

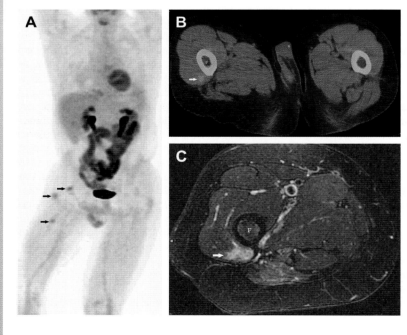

Fig. 8. Intramuscular metastases in a 61-year-old man who had esophageal cancer 10 months after preoperative chemoradiotherapy and surgical resection. (*A*) Whole-body maximum-intensity projection image shows focal increased FDG uptake in the soft tissues of the thigh (*arrows*). (*B*) Axial integrated PET-CT of the thighs shows a show focus of low-grade increased uptake (standardized uptake value 2.9) of FDG within the vastus lateralis muscle with no corresponding abnormality on CT (*arrow*). F, femur. (*C*) Axial T2-weighted MR image of the right thigh shows increased signal in the vastus lateralis muscle (*arrow*). The patient was asymptomatic, and resection revealed an intramuscular esophageal metastasis. F, femur.

been appropriately studied, and although the technique is often suggested as a potentially useful adjunct to the conventional work-up, it is not considered standard procedure. FDG-PET[68] and PET-CT[69] have been proposed for detecting and staging recurrent disease. Taking advantage of their high positive predictive value, they appear to be particularly useful in patients who have a high suspicion of recurrence based on other findings. Conversely, the negative predictive value is low, which requires an appropriate selection of patients being tested. Obviously, PET and PET-CT cannot be proposed as a screening tool in the postoperative follow-up.

SUMMARY

In summary, PET and integrated PET-CT are useful in the initial staging of patients who have esophageal and, to a lesser extent, gastric cancers being considered for curative surgical resection. Although PET has a limited role in the evaluation of the primary tumor and in the detection of locoregional nodal metastases, PET imaging is important in the detection of distant metastases. In this regard, PET and PET-CT can decrease inappropriate surgical resection mainly because of the detection of distant metastases not diagnosed by conventional evaluation. In addition, in patients who have suspected recurrent disease, PET and PET-CT can be helpful to detect sites of metastatic disease.

REFERENCES

1. Kamangar F, Dores GM, Anderson WF. Patterns of cancer incidence, mortality, and prevalence across five continents: defining priorities to reduce cancer disparities in different geographic regions of the world. J Clin Oncol 2006;24(14):2137–50.
2. Swisher SG, Ajani JA, Komaki R, et al. Long-term outcome of a phase II trial evaluating chemotherapy, chemoradiotherapy, and surgery for locoregionally advanced esophageal cancer. Int J Radiat Oncol Biol Phys 2003;57(1):120–7.
3. Swisher SG, Hunt KK, Holmes EC, et al. Changes in the surgical management of esophageal cancer from 1970 to 1993. Am J Surg 1995;169(6):609–14.
4. Berger AC, Farma J, Scott WJ, et al. Complete response to neoadjuvant chemoradiotherapy in esophageal carcinoma is associated with significantly improved survival. J Clin Oncol 2005;23(19):4330–7.
5. Moehler M, Lyros O, Gockel I, et al. Multidisciplinary management of gastric and gastroesophageal cancers. World J Gastroenterol 2008;14(24):3773–80.
6. Xi WD, Zhao C, Ren GS. Endoscopic ultrasonography in preoperative staging of gastric cancer: determination of tumor invasion depth, nodal involvement and surgical resectability. World J Gastroenterol 2003;9(2):254–7.
7. Puli SR, Batapati Krishna Reddy J, Bechtold ML, et al. How good is endoscopic ultrasound for TNM staging of gastric cancers? A meta-analysis and systematic review. World J Gastroenterol 2008;14(25):4011–9.
8. Puli SR, Reddy JB, Bechtold ML, et al. Staging accuracy of esophageal cancer by endoscopic ultrasound: a meta-analysis and systematic review. World J Gastroenterol 2008;14(10):1479–90.
9. Kwee RM, Kwee TC. Imaging in local staging of gastric cancer: a systematic review. J Clin Oncol 2007;25(15):2107–16.
10. Chen CY, Hsu JS, Wu DC, et al. Gastric cancer: preoperative local staging with 3D multi-detector row CT–correlation with surgical and histopathologic results. Radiology 2007;242(2):472–82.
11. Wakelin SJ, Deans C, Crofts TJ, et al. A comparison of computerised tomography, laparoscopic ultrasound and endoscopic ultrasound in the preoperative staging of oesophago-gastric carcinoma. Eur J Radiol 2002;41(2):161–7.
12. Wallace MB, Nietert PJ, Earle C, et al. An analysis of multiple staging management strategies for carcinoma of the esophagus: computed tomography, endoscopic ultrasound, positron emission tomography, and thoracoscopy/laparoscopy. Ann Thorac Surg 2002;74(4):1026–32.
13. van Vliet EP, Heijenbrok-Kal MH, Hunink MG, et al. Staging investigations for oesophageal cancer: a meta-analysis. Br J Cancer 2008;98(3):547–57.
14. Lowe VJ, Booya F, Fletcher JG, et al. Comparison of positron emission tomography, computed tomography, and endoscopic ultrasound in the initial staging of patients with esophageal cancer. Mol Imaging Biol 2005;7(6):422–30.
15. Pfau PR, Perlman SB, Stanko P, et al. The role and clinical value of EUS in a multimodality esophageal carcinoma staging program with CT and positron emission tomography. Gastrointest Endosc 2007;65(3):377–84.
16. Bar-Shalom R, Guralnik L, Tsalic M, et al. The additional value of PET/CT over PET in FDG imaging of oesophageal cancer. Eur J Nucl Med Mol Imaging 2005;32(8):918–24.
17. Schreurs LM, Pultrum BB, Koopmans KP, et al. Better assessment of nodal metastases by PET/CT fusion compared to side-by-side PET/CT in oesophageal cancer. Anticancer Res 2008;28(3B):1867–73.
18. Heye T, Kuntz C, Duxc M, et al. CT and endoscopic ultrasound in comparison to endoluminal MRI—preliminary results in staging gastric carcinoma. Eur J Radiol 2008 Mar 10. [Epub ahead of print].

19. Ozawa S, Imai Y, Suwa T, et al. What's new in imaging? New magnetic resonance imaging of esophageal cancer using an endoluminal surface coil and antibody-coated magnetite particles. Recent Results Cancer Res 2000;155:73–87.

20. Riddell AM, Davies DC, Allum WH, et al. High-resolution MRI in evaluation of the surgical anatomy of the esophagus and posterior mediastinum. AJR Am J Roentgenol 2007;188(1):W37–43.

21. Himeno S, Yasuda S, Shimada H, et al. Evaluation of esophageal cancer by positron emission tomography. Jpn J Clin Oncol 2002;32(9):340–6.

22. Kato H, Miyazaki T, Nakajima M, et al. The incremental effect of positron emission tomography on diagnostic accuracy in the initial staging of esophageal carcinoma. Cancer 2005;103(1):148–56.

23. Little SG, Rice TW, Bybel B, et al. Is FDG-PET indicated for superficial esophageal cancer? Eur J Cardiothorac Surg 2007;31(5):791–6.

24. Miyata H, Doki Y, Yasuda T, et al. Evaluation of clinical significance of 18F-fluorodeoxyglucose positron emission tomography in superficial squamous cell carcinomas of the thoracic esophagus. Dis Esophagus 2008;21(2):144–50.

25. American Joint Commission on Cancer. Esophagus. In: Greene FL PD, Fleming ID, Fritz AG, editors. American Joint Commission on Cancer, cancer staging manual. 6th edition. New York: Springer-Verlag; 2002. p. 301–46.

26. van Westreenen HL, Westerterp M, Bossuyt PM, et al. Systematic review of the staging performance of 18F-fluorodeoxyglucose positron emission tomography in esophageal cancer. J Clin Oncol 2004; 22(18):3805–12.

27. Block MI, Patterson GA, Sundaresan RS, et al. Improvement in staging of esophageal cancer with the addition of positron emission tomography. Ann Thorac Surg 1997;64(3):770–6 [discussion: 6–7].

28. Flamen P, Lerut A, Van Cutsem E, et al. Utility of positron emission tomography for the staging of patients with potentially operable esophageal carcinoma. J Clin Oncol 2000;18(18):3202–10.

29. Wren SM, Stijns P, Srinivas S. Positron emission tomography in the initial staging of esophageal cancer. Arch Surg 2002;137(9):1001–6 [discussion: 6–7].

30. Kluetz PG, Meltzer CC, Villemagne VL, et al. Combined PET/CT imaging in oncology. Impact on patient management. Clin Positron Imaging 2000;3(6):223–30.

31. Kole AC, Plukker JT, Nieweg OE, et al. Positron emission tomography for staging of oesophageal and gastroesophageal malignancy. Br J Cancer 1998;78(4):521–7.

32. Downey RJ, Akhurst T, Ilson D, et al. Whole body 18FDG-PET and the response of esophageal cancer to induction therapy: results of a prospective trial. J Clin Oncol 2003;21(3):428–32.

33. Westerterp M, van Westreenen HL, Reitsma JB, et al. Esophageal cancer: CT, endoscopic US, and FDG PET for assessment of response to neoadjuvant therapy—systematic review. Radiology 2005; 236(3):841–51.

34. Cerfolio RJ, Bryant AS. Maximum standardized uptake values on positron emission tomography of esophageal cancer predicts stage, tumor biology, and survival. Ann Thorac Surg 2006;82(2):391–4 [discussion: 4–5].

35. Rizk N, Downey RJ, Akhurst T, et al. Preoperative 18[F]-fluorodeoxyglucose positron emission tomography standardized uptake values predict survival after esophageal adenocarcinoma resection. Ann Thorac Surg 2006;81(3):1076–81.

36. Mamede M, Abreu ELP, Oliva MR, et al. FDG-PET/CT tumor segmentation-derived indices of metabolic activity to assess response to neoadjuvant therapy and progression-free survival in esophageal cancer: correlation with histopathology results. Am J Clin Oncol 2007;30(4):377–88.

37. Eloubeidi MA, Desmond R, Arguedas MR, et al. Prognostic factors for the survival of patients with esophageal carcinoma in the U.S.: the importance of tumor length and lymph node status. Cancer 2002;95(7):1434–43.

38. Griffiths EA, Brummell Z, Gorthi G, et al. Tumor length as a prognostic factor in esophageal malignancy: univariate and multivariate survival analyses. J Surg Oncol 2006;93(4):258–67.

39. Konski A, Doss M, Milestone B, et al. The integration of 18-fluoro-deoxy-glucose positron emission tomography and endoscopic ultrasound in the treatment-planning process for esophageal carcinoma. Int J Radiat Oncol Biol Phys 2005;61(4):1123–8.

40. Moureau-Zabotto L, Touboul E, Lerouge D, et al. Impact of CT and 18F-deoxyglucose positron emission tomography image fusion for conformal radiotherapy in esophageal carcinoma. Int J Radiat Oncol Biol Phys 2005;63(2):340–5.

41. Rice TW. Clinical staging of esophageal carcinoma. CT, EUS, and PET. Chest Surg Clin N Am 2000; 10(3):471–85.

42. Kneist W, Schreckenberger M, Bartenstein P, et al. Positron emission tomography for staging esophageal cancer: does it lead to a different therapeutic approach? World J Surg 2003;27(10):1105–12.

43. Heeren PA, Jager PL, Bongaerts F, et al. Detection of distant metastases in esophageal cancer with (18)F-FDG PET. J Nucl Med 2004;45(6):980–7.

44. Romagnuolo J, Scott J, Hawes RH, et al. Helical CT versus EUS with fine needle aspiration for celiac nodal assessment in patients with esophageal cancer. Gastrointest Endosc 2002;55(6):648–54.

45. Parmar KS, Zwischenberger JB, Reeves AL, et al. Clinical impact of endoscopic ultrasound-guided fine needle aspiration of celiac axis lymph nodes (M1a disease) in esophageal cancer. Ann Thorac Surg 2002;73(3):916–20 [discussion: 20–1].

46. Eloubeidi MA, Wallace MB, Hoffman BJ, et al. Predictors of survival for esophageal cancer patients with and without celiac axis lymphadenopathy: impact of staging endosonography. Ann Thorac Surg 2001;72(1):212–9 [discussion: 9–0].

47. Katsoulis IE, Wong WL, Mattheou AK, et al. Fluorine-18 fluorodeoxyglucose positron emission tomography in the preoperative staging of thoracic oesophageal and gastro-oesophageal junction cancer: a prospective study. Int J Surg 2007;5(6):399–403.

48. Meyers BF, Downey RJ, Decker PA, et al. The utility of positron emission tomography in staging of potentially operable carcinoma of the thoracic esophagus: results of the American College of Surgeons Oncology Group Z0060 trial. J Thorac Cardiovasc Surg 2007;133(3):738–45.

49. Flanagan FL, Dehdashti F, Siegel BA, et al. Staging of esophageal cancer with 18F-fluorodeoxyglucose positron emission tomography. AJR Am J Roentgenol 1997;168(2):417–24.

50. Luketich JD, Friedman DM, Weigel TL, et al. Evaluation of distant metastases in esophageal cancer: 100 consecutive positron emission tomography scans. Ann Thorac Surg 1999;68(4):1133–6 [discussion: 6–7].

51. Liberale G, Van Laethem JL, Gay F, et al. The role of PET scan in the preoperative management of oesophageal cancer. Eur J Surg Oncol 2004;30(9):942–7.

52. van Westreenen HL, Westerterp M, Sloof GW, et al. Limited additional value of positron emission tomography in staging oesophageal cancer. Br J Surg 2007;94(12):1515–20.

53. Law SY, Fok M, Wong J. Pattern of recurrence after oesophageal resection for cancer: clinical implications. Br J Surg 1996;83(1):107–11.

54. van Lanschot JJ, Tilanus HW, Voormolen MH, et al. Recurrence pattern of oesophageal carcinoma after limited resection does not support wide local excision with extensive lymph node dissection. Br J Surg 1994;81(9):1320–3.

55. Hsieh C, Chow K, Fahn H, et al. Prognostic significance of HER-2/neu overexpression in stage I adenocarcinoma of lung. Ann Thorac Surg 1998;66:1159–64.

56. Raoul JL, Le Prise E, Meunier B, et al. Combined radiochemotherapy for postoperative recurrence of oesophageal cancer. Gut 1995;37(2):174–6.

57. Flamen P, Van Cutsem E, Lerut A, et al. Positron emission tomography for assessment of the response to induction radiochemotherapy in locally advanced oesophageal cancer. Ann Oncol 2002;13(3):361–8.

58. Weber WA, Ott K, Becker K, et al. Prediction of response to preoperative chemotherapy in adenocarcinomas of the esophagogastric junction by metabolic imaging. J Clin Oncol 2001;19(12):3058–65.

59. Cerfolio RJ, Bryant AS, Ohja B, et al. The accuracy of endoscopic ultrasonography with fine-needle aspiration, integrated positron emission tomography with computed tomography, and computed tomography in restaging patients with esophageal cancer after neoadjuvant chemoradiotherapy. J Thorac Cardiovasc Surg 2005;129(6):1232–41.

60. Bruzzi JF, Swisher SG, Truong MT, et al. Detection of interval distant metastases: clinical utility of integrated CT-PET imaging in patients with esophageal carcinoma after neoadjuvant therapy. Cancer 2007;109(1):125–34.

61. Bruzzi JF, Truong MT, Macapinlac H, et al. Integrated CT-PET imaging of esophageal cancer: unexpected and unusual distribution of distant organ metastases. Curr Probl Diagn Radiol 2007;36(1):21–9.

62. Stahl A, Ott K, Weber WA, et al. FDG PET imaging of locally advanced gastric carcinomas: correlation with endoscopic and histopathological findings. Eur J Nucl Med Mol Imaging 2003;30(2):288–95.

63. Yoshioka T, Yamaguchi K, Kubota K, et al. Evaluation of 18F-FDG PET in patients with a, metastatic, or recurrent gastric cancer. J Nucl Med 2003;44(5):690–9.

64. McAteer D, Wallis F, Couper G, et al. Evaluation of 18F-FDG positron emission tomography in gastric and oesophageal carcinoma. Br J Radiol 1999;72(858):525–9.

65. Yun M, Lim JS, Noh SH, et al. Lymph node staging of gastric cancer using (18)F-FDG PET: a comparison study with CT. J Nucl Med 2005;46(10):1582–8.

66. Tian J, Chen L, Wei B, et al. The value of vesicant 18F-fluorodeoxyglucose positron emission tomography (18F-FDG PET) in gastric malignancies. Nucl Med Commun 2004;25(8):825–31.

67. Chen J, Cheong JH, Yun MJ, et al. Improvement in preoperative staging of gastric adenocarcinoma with positron emission tomography. Cancer 2005;103(11):2383–90.

68. De Potter T, Flamen P, Van Cutsem E, et al. Whole-body PET with FDG for the diagnosis of recurrent gastric cancer. Eur J Nucl Med Mol Imaging 2002;29(4):525–9.

69. Park MJ, Lee WJ, Lim HK, et al. Detecting recurrence of gastric cancer: the value of FDG PET/CT. Abdom Imaging 2008.

FDG-PET and PET/CT in Colorectal Cancer

Max Lonneux, MD, PhD

KEYWORDS

• PET-CT • FDG • Colorectal cancer • Recurrence • Staging

Colorectal cancer (CRC) is the second most common cause of cancer-related deaths in Western countries. Treatment relies on curative surgery. For rectal cancer, combined approaches with adjuvant radio-chemotherapy plus surgery have proven effective. However, even after a well-conducted curative-intent treatment, 30% to 50% of patients experience tumor relapse.

Accurate initial staging of CRC is mandatory for optimal therapeutic planning. As a whole-body imaging technique, fluorodeoxyglucose (FDG) positron emission tomography (PET) and PET-CT have the unique capability of providing staging for the tumor (T) stage, nodal (N) stage, and metastatic (M) stage in a single imaging session. This article covers the use of FDG PET and PET-CT scanning for the initial staging, and for the detection and staging of tumor relapse. The particular aspect of treatment monitoring is covered in a separate contribution elsewhere in this issue.

PRACTICAL CONSIDERATIONS

Several specific considerations apply when using FDG PET-CT for colorectal cancer imaging. First, physiologic bowel uptake is observed in many patients. Usually this uptake is faint, homogeneous, and predominant in the right colon. However, in some cases, it can be very intense and spotty, mimicking pathologic uptake. Bowel uptake is mainly related to motility, but can also result from lymphoid tissue activation, especially in younger patients. Moreover, numerous benign diseases, such as enterocolitis, inflammatory bowel diseases, and diverticulitis, can lead to increased and spotty bowel uptake. Careful

evaluation of the uptake pattern is mandatory to avoid false-positive interpretations. The CT signs (in case of PET-CT examination) can also be helpful.[1] Full bowel preparation (ie, cleansing using an iso-osmotic solution given the day before the procedure) has been shown to significantly decrease the physiologic bowel uptake.[2] However, such an approach has not been widely implemented in clinical centers.

Second, a quick look at the histology of the primary tumor is useful because mucinous adenocarcinomas are poorly avid for FDG. Indeed, given a low cellularity and high fatty component, their overall FDG uptake is low and yields to a very limited sensitivity. When interpreting a PET scan, one should be aware of the histopathological subtype and, if mucoid, then one should clearly state on the report that there is a high probability of false-negative findings.[3]

Third, the liver is the main metastatic organ in colon cancer and the normal liver parenchyma can display a rather high uptake of FDG, impeding the visualization of small liver metastases. Normal liver cells can further metabolize FDG after the initial phosphorylation step. In time, the tracer is dephosphorylated and leaves the hepatocyte, while remaining inside the tumor cell. Thus, a longer delay between injection of the tracer and the image acquisition can be helpful. This allows for a higher tumor-to-liver ratio (ie, a higher tumor uptake together with a decreased normal liver uptake). Indeed, recent research has shown that FDG PET scans 120 minutes after injection found hepatic lesions that were missed in 17% of images obtained 90 minutes after injection.[4] This is an interesting finding, especially when one considers

Department of Nuclear Medicine, Molecular Imaging and Experimental Radiotherapy Unit, Cliniques Universitaires Saint-Luc, Avenue Hippocrate 10, B-1200, UCL, Brussels, Belgium
E-mail address: max.lonneux@uclouvain.be

PET Clin 3 (2008) 147–153
doi:10.1016/j.cpet.2008.08.004

that the clinical standard in many centers is to image patients as soon as 60 minutes after injection.

Finally, forced diuresis by intravenous hydration with or without diuretics should be considered for rectal cancer imaging. Again, delayed imaging would allow for a complete bladder voiding and dilution of the excreted activity, thereby increasing the signal-to-noise ratio in the pelvic area.

INCIDENTAL COLORECTAL HOT SPOTS

Incidental FDG hot spots have been reported in up to 3% of the patients having an FDG PET-CT procedure. In up to 78% of the cases, hot spots correspond to an actual lesion, either benign (hyperplastic polyps, ulcers, adenomas, hemorrhoids) or malignant (adenocarcinomas, villous tumors).[5–8] FDG uptake is more intense with increasing grade of colonic adenomas.[9] Therefore, incidental hot spots seen on FDG PET scans must be taken seriously and further exploration (ie, colonoscopy) is mandatory.

INITIAL DIAGNOSIS AND PRETHERAPEUTIC STAGING OF COLORECTAL CANCER

The current guidelines do not recommend FDG PET-CT for the initial preoperative staging of CRC. Despite a high sensitivity for the primary tumor as well as for distant metastases detection, FDG PET was initially shown to have a marginal impact on patient management, compared with preoperative abdominopelvic CT. The sensitivity for detection of locoregional lymph node metastases is low because lymph nodes are usually close to the primary tumor and cannot be differentiated from the primary tumor.[10–12] CT might help in the detection of small lymph nodes adjacent to the primary but it is still difficult to classify a small lymph node as metastatic if its uptake cannot be clearly separated from the primary, which is often bulky.[13] Interestingly, Inoue and colleagues[14] recently reported that they were able to increase the detection rate of lymph nodes on FDG PET by applying an iterative algorithm for image interpretation. After three iterations, the sensitivity increased from 51.3% (visual analysis) to 79.4%. This kind of approach is interesting but relies on quite complex image processing and has to be implemented in a clinical environment.

As a pretherapeutic staging modality, FDG PET mainly alters patient management by detecting distant metastases in cases where conventional imaging methods were either inconclusive or false negative. Compared with CT, PET-CT provides similar diagnostic performance for hepatic metastases detection. However, PET is more accurate for the detection of extrahepatic sites, such as periportal lymph nodes, para-aortic lymph nodes, and peritoneal carcinomatosis.[15,16] PET is also able to detect synchronous colonic lesions when it is impossible to pass through the primary lesion with the endoscope.[12] In terms of patient management, some studies indicate that FDG PET does modify the patient management,[12–15] but other studies report that PET is no better than multidetector CT.[17] Differences observed might be partly due to differences in study population. Indeed, in the (positive for PET) study of Park and colleagues, patients were included on the basis of either elevated carcinoembryonic antigen (CEA) (equal to or above 10 ng/mL) or equivocal CT. Thus, compared with patients from a general unselected population, patients with equivocal CT were more likely to obtain an accurate restaging with PET.

Recent studies using combined PET-CT colonography (ie, with dedicated colon preparation and image-acquisition protocols) have reported that, in staging colon cancer, combined PET-CT colonography delivers accuracies superior to CT alone and to CT plus PET performed separately.[18,19] A combined PET-CT colonography procedure requires adequate colon cleansing and takes a little bit longer than conventional PET-CT, but has the advantage of providing a full staging report in a single procedure. Veit-Haibach and colleagues[18] reported an 80% sensitivity for N stage and a 100% sensitivity for M detection in a pilot study of 47 patients. They also reported that PET-CT colonography affected the therapy decisions in 4 patients (9%). This technique has also shown good results to assess the colon proximal to an obstructive CRC.

Should PET be a part of the standard initial staging of CRC? Somehow conflicting results on the impact of FDG PET-CT in the initial preoperative staging of CRC coexist in the literature. In the United States, PET is reimbursed if "staging is uncertain following conventional imaging, and if the clinical management of the patient may differ according to the stage."[20] PET-CT is not presently part of the international guidelines for CRC initial staging.[21,22] However, it is recommended when CT is inconclusive or equivocal in advanced CRC.[23] This looks like a fair assumption and should be considered as the current guideline. New technical approaches, such as PET-CT colonography, still need more investigations, especially in terms of cost-efficacy.

Some studies have focused specifically on rectal cancer, and have shown a significant percentage (around 30%) of tumor stage change with FDG PET. Recently, Davey and colleagues[24] conducted a prospective study to assess the impact of FDG

PET on patient management and reported that the management was altered in 10 of 83 (12%) patients. The TNM stage was changed in 31% of patients, with upstage and downstage occurring in almost equal proportions. Change in management seems more frequent (27%) in low rectal cancers, as reported by Gearhart and colleagues,[25] in particular by detecting positive inguinal lymph nodes that are a characteristic metastatic site of low rectal tumors. Rectal cancer staging raises the specific questions of both tumor volume delineation (for radiotherapy treatment planning) and of monitoring of tumor response to preoperative chemoradiation, which is the standard of care for locally advanced tumors. Metabolic imaging using PET-CT can identify tumor subvolumes that are more aggressive and should receive higher doses of radiation. A high FDG uptake before therapy is indeed related to reduced overall survival.[26] Modern radiotherapy techniques, such as intensity-modulated radiation therapy, allow for precise dose sculpting and the concept of "biological target volume" has recently emerged, based on the use of PET for tumor volume delineation. Also, FDG PET accurately measures the response to chemoradiation, while both CT and MR imaging have consistently failed to discriminate responders from nonresponders. Late (4 to 5 weeks after the end of chemoradiation) or even very early (as soon as 12 days after the start of chemoradiation) FDG PET correlates with the histopathological tumor regression grade.[27,28] It is therefore likely that FDG PET-CT will soon become a standard for the staging of locally advanced rectal tumors, both because it can change the TNM stage, and because it can be used for tumor volume delineation and for (early) assessment of response. Such a case is illustrated in **Fig. 1**.

DETECTION OF TUMOR RECURRENCE

There is a general agreement that systematic postoperative surveillance of CRC patients is useful because it has been demonstrated that early treatment of tumor relapse improves patients' prognoses.[29] A recent prospective trial showed that an intensive follow-up scheme, adding abdominal/chest imaging and colonoscopy to CEA monitoring, yielded a higher rate of resectable recurrences, and improved survival in patients with stage II or rectal tumors.[30]

Follow-up based on sequential CEA dosage raises the question of identifying the site of relapse once the marker level is found abnormal. FDG PET-CT is a very sensitive imaging technique in that setting. In a study of 50 patients, Flamen and colleagues[31] indeed showed that PET detected tumor relapse in 79% of cases and led to

curative-intent surgery in 14 of 50 patients (28%). More recently, a randomized controlled trial has shed light on the potential use of FDG PET as a surveillance imaging technique in CRC patients. One hundred and thirty patients operated on with curative intent were randomly assigned to either conventional follow-up or to conventional-plus-PET follow-up. Recurrence was diagnosed in 44 of 130 patients, 23 in the PET group and 21 in the conventional group. The time interval from baseline to recurrence detection was significantly reduced in the PET group compared with the conventional group (12.1 months vs 15.4 months, $P = .01$). Not only did PET allow for an earlier diagnosis of relapse, but the rate of successful curative intent surgery (R0) was significantly higher in the PET group: Ten out of 23 patients could be treated with curative intent, versus 2 out of 21 in the conventional group ($P<.01$) (**Fig. 2**).[32] Also, CEA is not a good indicator of tumor activity in all patients, and clinical and follow-up imaging workup can be the first sign of possible recurrence. Even in patients with a normal CEA level but with a clinical suspicion of recurrence, the positive predictive value of FDG PET is very high (85%).[33] There is also evidence supporting the use of FDG PET-CT for the detection of loco-regional relapse, especially at the pelvic level where fibrotic or scar tissue is difficult to discriminate from recurrence on CT or MR image.[34] These data clearly suggest that FDG PET should be used very early in the evaluation of patients with treated CRC, and even maybe as a systematic surveillance technique in high-risk patients, especially during the first 2 years after initial treatment because 80% of recurrences occur during that period.

STAGING OF RECURRENCE AND ASSESSMENT OF RESECTABILITY

The most common clinical application of FDG PET-CT is in the assessment of resectability of a known tumor recurrence, diagnosed by so-called "first-line" imaging techniques (liver ultrasound, follow-up CT). Given the limited availability of FDG PET-CT even nowadays, recurrence is often diagnosed by other means and PET is ordered for staging purposes. Strong evidence in the literature supports the use of FDG PET or PET-CT in that setting. The liver is the main site of CRC recurrence. Metastasectomy (either alone or combined with chemotherapy, chemoembolization, and radiofrequency ablation) is indicated provided the disease is limited to the liver. FDG PET has consistently outperformed CT in detecting extrahepatic disease, yielding a more accurate patient selection for liver surgery, an improved resectability rate, and prolonged survival in

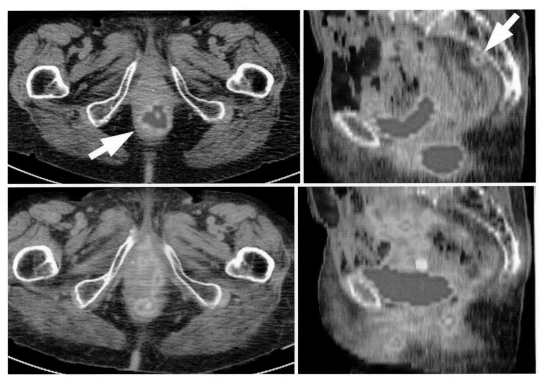

Fig. 1. Pre- and posttherapeutic FDG PET-CT of a 90-year-old woman with anorectal cancer. (*Top*) Baseline PET-CT showing a high uptake in the primary tumor (primary tumor standardized uptake value 12), and a positive lymph node in the presacral basin (*arrows*). (*Bottom*) FDG PET-CT obtained 11 weeks after completion of radiotherapy (60 Gy) delivered on the primary tumor and PET-positive lymph nodes. There is a good metabolic response at the primary tumor level (primary tumor standardized uptake value drops to 3.1). The large reduction in the primary tumor standardized uptake value at the primary level (−75%) together with the complete disappearance of the presacral hot spots classify the patient as responder.

patients with limited disease on PET.[35–40] Two meta-analyses reported that FDG PET had a higher sensitivity/specificity for detecting extrahepatic disease (91.5% to 95.4% vs 60.9% to 91.1%) compared with CT[41] or to MR imaging (sensitivity of 94.6% vs 75.8%, respectively).[42] In a recent publication, Wiering and colleagues[43] reported on 203 patients with liver metastases from CRC accrued between 1995 and 2003, and compared those staged without (n = 100) and with FDG-PET (n = 103). The number of patients with futile surgery (ie, in whom at laparotomy the extent of disease was too large for a curative-intent resection) was 28% in the group without PET, compared with 19.4% in the group with PET used for staging. Interestingly, 10 patients (10%) from the group without PET showed unsuspected extrahepatic abdominal disease at laparotomy, versus only 2 patients from the group with PET, illustrating the higher sensitivity of FDG PET to depict extrahepatic tumor seeding.

Overall, FDG PET significantly alters the management of patients with recurrent CRC in approximately 30% of cases.[44] With the introduction of combined PET-CT, the overall diagnostic performance has even been increased. The number of equivocal findings on PET (due to physiologic bowel uptake, urinary tract interference, or poor spatial localization of hot spots) has been reduced by 50%, and the staging accuracy improves from 78% to 89%.[45] Moreover, PET-CT with contrast-enhanced CT (ie, full diagnostic CT) further adds pertinent diagnostic information to classical PET-CT (without CT contrast injection). In a series of 54 patients included for restaging CRC, PET-CT added correct diagnostic findings in 27 patients (50%) compared with contrast-enhanced CT alone. However, PET with contrast-enhanced CT (ie, the CT part of PET-CT being full diagnostic with contrast injection) added diagnostic information in 39 patients compared with PET-CT (72%), and altered the therapeutic

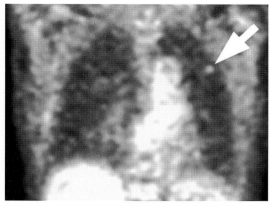

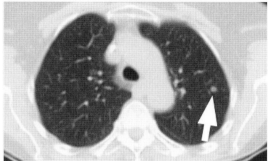

Fig. 2. A 69-year-old woman operated on 16 months before for a T3N2 sigmoid adenocarcinoma, presenting with an increasing CEA level (12 ng/mL). Whole-body FDG PET-CT shows a hot spot in the upper part of the left lung (*top, arrow, coronal view*), corresponding to a 6-mm nodule on the low-dose CT (*bottom, arrow*). This turned out to be a lung metastasis.

management in 23 patients. The incremental value of contrast enhanced PET-CT was mainly a correct segmental localization of liver metastases, which is important information as far as treatment planning is concerned.[46]

A new whole-body procedure, whole-body MR imaging, has been recently developed and is presented as a potential challenger to whole-body FDG PET-CT for staging of cancer. The initial clinical experience comparing whole-body MR imaging and PET-CT in CRC patients has been recently published. Whole-body MR imaging detected more hepatic metastases than PET-CT (27 vs 23 lesions), but each technique classified the same number of patients[15] as having liver metastases. PET-CT depicted more lung metastases (25 vs 19 lesions) in more patients (7 vs 5). Performances of both techniques were equivalent for detecting bone and peritoneal metastases.[47]

RISK STRATIFICATION

Beyond its huge potential as a cancer-detecting tool, PET-CT imaging further allows for the in vivo characterization of tumor biology. High FDG uptake measured by PET correlates with poorer outcome (reduced survival, reduced disease-free survival) of solid tumors, such as breast cancers.[48] Such a prognostic value of FDG uptake by recurrent CRC has been evaluated by de Geus-Oei and colleagues[49] In a series of 152 patients with metastatic CRC (67 operated, 85 treated with chemotherapy), they were able to show that the FDG uptake (as measured by standardized uptake values [SUV]) was a significant and independent predictor of the overall survival. The median survival was 32 months in the group with low FDG-uptake tumors (SUV < 4.26) and 19 months in the group with highly metabolic tumors (SUV > 4.26). Accordingly, the 2-year and 3-year survival rates were reduced in the high-uptake group: 37% and 28% versus 59% and 45% in the low-uptake group. Riedl and colleagues[50] measured the FDG uptake in liver metastases before surgical resection in a group of 90 patients. They showed that for highly metabolic tumors, the median survival after surgery was reduced. These preliminary results pave the way for a more subtle patient selection for adjuvant treatment after surgery (ie, combining chemotherapeutic and biological agents in patients with highly metabolic tumors).

SUMMARY

Strong scientific evidence supports the use of whole-body FDG PET-CT in the assessment of suspected recurrence of CRC or in the pretherapeutic staging before liver (or lung) metastasectomy. FDG PET-CT should be considered a standard of care in these clinical situations. Recent results emphasize the use of PET as a first-line imaging procedure for the follow-up of high-risk patients (typically, stage III-IV CRC), even as a systematic surveillance procedure.

New potential indications are the baseline pretherapeutic staging of rectal cancers, especially in the framework of modern multimodal therapies (neoadjuvant chemoradiation).

REFERENCES

1. Prabhakar HB, Sahani DV, Fischman AJ, et al. Bowel hot spots at PET-CT. Radiographics 2007;27:145–59.
2. Miraldi F, Vesselle H, Faulhaber PF, et al. Elimination of artifactual accumulation of FDG in PET imaging of colorectal cancer. Clin Nucl Med 1998;23:3–7.
3. Berger KL, Nicholson SA, Dehdashti F, et al. FDG PET evaluation of mucinous neoplasms: correlation of FDG uptake with histopathologic features. AJR Am J Roentgenol 2000;174:1005–8.

4. Kuker RA, Mesoloras G, Gulec SA. Optimization of FDG-PET/CT imaging protocol for evaluation of patients with primary and metastatic liver disease. Int Semin Surg Oncol 2007;4:17.

5. Agress HJ, Cooper BZ. Detection of clinically unexpected malignant and premalignant tumors with whole-body FDG PET: histopathologic comparison. Radiology 2004;230:417–22.

6. Drenth JP, Nagengast FM, Oyen WJ. Evaluation of (pre-)malignant colonic abnormalities: endoscopic validation of FDG-PET findings. Eur J Nucl Med 2001;28:1766–9.

7. Israel O, Yefremov N, Bar-Shalom R, et al. PET/CT detection of unexpected gastrointestinal foci of 18F-FDG uptake: incidence, localization patterns, and clinical significance. J Nucl Med 2005;46:758–62.

8. Kamel EM, Thumshirn M, Truninger K, et al. Significance of incidental 18F-FDG accumulations in the gastrointestinal tract in PET/CT: correlation with endoscopic and histopathologic results. J Nucl Med 2004;45:1804–10.

9. van Kouwen MC, Nagengast FM, Jansen JB, et al. 2-(18F)-fluoro-2-deoxy-D-glucose positron emission tomography detects clinical relevant adenomas of the colon: a prospective study. J Clin Oncol 2005;23:3713–7.

10. Abdel-Nabi H, Doerr RJ, Lamonica DM, et al. Staging of primary colorectal carcinomas with fluorine-18 fluorodeoxyglucose whole-body PET: correlation with histopathologic and CT findings. Radiology 1998;206:755–60.

11. Kantorova I, Lipska L, Belohlavek O, et al. Routine (18)F-FDG PET preoperative staging of colorectal cancer: comparison with conventional staging and its impact on treatment decision making. J Nucl Med 2003;44:1784–8.

12. Llamas-Elvira JM, Rodriguez-Fernandez A, Gutier-rez-Sainz J, et al. Fluorine-18 fluorodeoxyglucose PET in the preoperative staging of colorectal cancer. Eur J Nucl Med Mol Imaging 2007;34:859–67.

13. Shin SS, Jeong YY, Min JJ, et al. Preoperative staging of colorectal cancer: CT vs. integrated FDG PET/CT. Abdom Imaging 2008;33:270–7.

14. Inoue K, Sato T, Kitamura H, et al. Diagnosis supporting algorithm for lymph node metastases from colorectal carcinoma on 18F-FDG PET/CT. Ann Nucl Med 2008;22:41–8.

15. Park IJ, Kim HC, Yu CS, et al. Efficacy of PET/CT in the accurate evaluation of primary colorectal carcinoma. Eur J Surg Oncol 2006;32:941–7.

16. Selzner M, Hany TF, Wildbrett P, et al. Does the novel PET/CT imaging modality impact on the treatment of patients with metastatic colorectal cancer of the liver? Ann Surg 2004;240:1027–34 [discussion: 1035–6].

17. Furukawa H, Ikuma H, Seki A, et al. Positron emission tomography scanning is not superior to whole body multidetector helical computed tomography in the preoperative staging of colorectal cancer. Gut 2006;55:1007–11.

18. Veit-Haibach P, Kuehle CA, Beyer T, et al. Diagnostic accuracy of colorectal cancer staging with whole-body PET/CT colonography. JAMA 2006;296:2590–600.

19. Nagata K, Ota Y, Okawa T, et al. PET/CT colonography for the preoperative evaluation of the colon proximal to the obstructive colorectal cancer. Dis Colon Rectum 2008;51:882–90.

20. Herbertson RA, Lee ST, Tebbutt N, et al. The expanding role of PET technology in the management of patients with colorectal cancer. Ann Oncol 2007;18:1774–81.

21. Fletcher JW, Djulbegovic B, Soares HP, et al. Recommendations on the use of 18F-FDG PET in oncology. J Nucl Med 2008;49:480–508.

22. Van Cutsem EJ, Oliveira J. Colon cancer: ESMO clinical recommendations for diagnosis, adjuvant treatment and follow-up. Ann Oncol 2008;19(Suppl 2):ii29–30.

23. Van Cutsem EJ, Oliveira J. Advanced colorectal cancer: ESMO clinical recommendations for diagnosis, treatment and follow-up. Ann Oncol 2008;19(Suppl 2):ii33–4.

24. Davey K, Heriot AG, Mackay J, et al. The impact of 18-fluorodeoxyglucose positron emission tomography–computed tomography on the staging and management of primary rectal cancer. Dis Colon Rectum 2008;51:997–1003.

25. Gearhart SL, Frassica D, Rosen R, et al. Improved staging with pretreatment positron emission tomography/computed tomography in low rectal cancer. Ann Surg Oncol 2006;13:397–404.

26. Calvo FA, Domper M, Matute R, et al. 18F-FDG positron emission tomography staging and restaging in rectal cancer treated with preoperative chemoradiation. Int J Radiat Oncol Biol Phys 2004;58:528–35.

27. Capirci C, Rampin L, Erba PA, et al. Sequential FDG-PET/CT reliably predicts response of locally advanced rectal cancer to neo-adjuvant chemo-radiation therapy. Eur J Nucl Med Mol Imaging 2007;34:1583–93.

28. Cascini GL, Avallone A, Delrio P, et al. 18F-FDG PET is an early predictor of pathologic tumor response to preoperative radiochemotherapy in locally advanced rectal cancer. J Nucl Med 2006;47:1241–8.

29. Renehan AG, Egger M, Saunders MP, et al. Impact on survival of intensive follow up after curative resection for colorectal cancer: systematic review and meta-analysis of randomised trials. BMJ 2002;324:813.

30. Rodriguez-Moranta F, Salo J, Arcusa A, et al. Postoperative surveillance in patients with colorectal cancer who have undergone curative resection:

a prospective, multicenter, randomized, controlled trial. J Clin Oncol 2006;24:386–93.

31. Flamen P, Hoekstra OS, Homans F, et al. Unexplained rising carcinoembryonic antigen (CEA) in the postoperative surveillance of colorectal cancer: the utility of positron emission tomography (PET). Eur J Cancer 2001;37:862–9.

32. Sobhani I, Tiret E, Lebtahi R, et al. Early detection of recurrence by 18FDG-PET in the follow-up of patients with colorectal cancer. Br J Cancer 2008; 98:875–80.

33. Sarikaya I, Bloomston M, Povoski SP, et al. FDG-PET scan in patients with clinically and/or radiologically suspicious colorectal cancer recurrence but normal CEA. World J Surg Oncol 2007;5:64.

34. Strauss LG, Clorius JH, Schlag P, et al. Recurrence of colorectal tumors: PET evaluation. Radiology 1989;170:329–32.

35. Arulampalam T, Costa D, Visvikis D, et al. The impact of FDG-PET on the management algorithm for recurrent colorectal cancer. Eur J Nucl Med 2001; 28:1758–65.

36. Kalff V, Hicks RJ, Ware RE, et al. The clinical impact of (18)F-FDG PET in patients with suspected or confirmed recurrence of colorectal cancer: a prospective study. J Nucl Med 2002;43:492–9.

37. Kong G, Jackson C, Koh DM, et al. The use of (18)F-FDG PET/CT in colorectal liver metastases—comparison with CT and liver MRI. Eur J Nucl Med Mol Imaging 2008;35:1323–9.

38. Lonneux M, Reffad AM, Detry R, et al. FDG-PET improves the staging and selection of patients with recurrent colorectal cancer. Eur J Nucl Med Mol Imaging 2002;29:915–21.

39. Ruers TJ, Langenhoff BS, Neeleman N, et al. Value of positron emission tomography with [F-18]fluorodeoxyglucose in patients with colorectal liver metastases: a prospective study. J Clin Oncol 2002;20: 388–95.

40. Strasberg SM, Dehdashti F, Siegel BA, et al. Survival of patients evaluated by FDG-PET before hepatic resection for metastatic colorectal carcinoma: a prospective database study. Ann Surg 2001;233: 293–9.

41. Wiering B, Krabbe PF, Jager GJ, et al. The impact of fluor-18-deoxyglucose-positron emission tomography in the management of colorectal liver metastases. Cancer 2005;104:2658–70.

42. Bipat S, van Leeuwen MS, Comans EF, et al. Colorectal liver metastases: CT, MR imaging, and PET for diagnosis–meta-analysis. Radiology 2005;237: 123–31.

43. Wiering B, Krabbe PF, Dekker HM, et al. The role of FDG-PET in the selection of patients with colorectal liver metastases. Ann Surg Oncol 2007;14:771–9.

44. Huebner RH, Park KC, Shepherd JE, et al. A meta-analysis of the literature for whole-body FDG PET detection of recurrent colorectal cancer. J Nucl Med 2000;41:1177–89.

45. Cohade C, Osman M, Leal J, et al. Direct comparison of (18)F-FDG PET and PET/CT in patients with colorectal carcinoma. J Nucl Med 2003;44: 1797–803.

46. Soyka JD, Veit-Haibach P, Strobel K, et al. Staging pathways in recurrent colorectal carcinoma: Is contrast-enhanced 18F-FDG PET/CT the diagnostic tool of choice? J Nucl Med 2008;49:354–61.

47. Squillaci E, Manenti G, Mancino S, et al. Staging of colon cancer: whole-body MRI vs. whole-body PET-CT—initial clinical experience. Abdom Imaging 2008.

48. Emmering J, Krak NC, Van der Hoeven JJ, et al. Preoperative [18F] FDG-PET after chemotherapy in locally advanced breast cancer: prognostic value as compared with histopathology. Ann Oncol 2008; 19:1573–7.

49. de Geus-Oei LF, Wiering B, Krabbe PF, et al. FDG-PET for prediction of survival of patients with metastatic colorectal carcinoma. Ann Oncol 2006;17:1650–5.

50. Riedl CC, Akhurst T, Larson S, et al. 18F-FDG PET scanning correlates with tissue markers of poor prognosis and predicts mortality for patients after liver resection for colorectal metastases. J Nucl Med 2007;48:771–5.

PET and PET/CT for Pancreatic Malignancies

Dominique Delbeke, MD, PhD, FACNP*, William H. Martin, MD

KEYWORDS

- Pancreatic carcinoma • FDG PET
- Cystic pancreatic lesions

Pancreatic ductal adenocarcinoma is the most common type of pancreatic cancer and arises from the pancreatic ducts. It is the third most common malignant tumor of the gastrointestinal tract and the fifth leading cause of cancer-related mortality accounting for 5% of cancer-related deaths in the United States.[1] Most tumors arise in the head of the pancreas, and patients present with bile duct obstruction, pain, and jaundice. Only 10% to 30% of pancreatic carcinomas are resectable at the time of presentation, the 5-year survival is 18% to 20%, and median survival is 17 to 21 months.[2] Patients with locally advanced nonmetastatic disease have a median survival of 6 to 10 months. Pancreatic carcinoma commonly metastasizes to the liver and patients with metastatic disease have a median survival of 3 to 6 months.

Carcinoma of the ampulla of Vater may be difficult to differentiate from those arising from the head of the pancreas. Ampullary carcinomas have a better prognosis than pancreatic carcinoma because they cause symptomatic biliary obstruction and are diagnosed earlier in the course of the disease.

Acinar cell carcinomas comprise no more than 1% to 2% of all pancreatic cancer, and the prognosis is as poor as for ductal adenocarcinoma.

Cystic neoplasms can arise in the pancreas and differentiation of benign from malignant is critical.

Islet cell tumors and other neuroendocrine (NE) tumors make up a small fraction of all pancreatic neoplasms and are most often located in the body and tail of the pancreas. They are usually slow-growing tumors and are associated with endocrine abnormalities. Endocrine pancreatic tumors include carcinoid tumors, insulinoma that is

benign in 90% of patients, gastrinoma, vipoma, and glucagoma that are metastatic at diagnosis in 60% to 80% of patients. The NE tumors will be addressed in another article.

Some of these tumors are associated with elevated serum levels of tumor markers that can be helpful for the diagnosis and surveillance of these patients, such as CA 19-9 for surveillance of patients with pancreatic ductal adenocarcinoma, as well as various peptides for islet cell neoplasms.

The diagnostic issues include early detection, differentiation of malignant from benign tumors (lesion characterization), staging for resection that includes lesion localization, evaluation of proximity to vessels, invasion of adjacent structures, metastasis to regional lymph nodes and distant sites, and assessment of therapeutic response.

Various imaging modalities are available to achieve these goals including ultrasound (US), computed tomography (CT), magnetic resonance imaging (MR imaging), and functional imaging using radiopharmaceuticals (nuclear medicine). Tomographic imaging for functional radioisotopic studies can be performed using single-photon emission tomography technique (SPECT) if the radiopharmaceutical is a single photon emitter, and positron emission tomography technique (PET) if the radiopharmaceutical is a positron emitter.

ANATOMIC IMAGING MODALITIES

The suspicion for pancreatic cancer is often raised when either a pancreatic mass or dilatation of the biliary or pancreatic ducts are detected by US or CT.

Department of Radiology and Radiological Sciences, Vanderbilt University Medical Center, 21st Avenue South and Garland, Nashville, TN 37232-2675, USA
* Corresponding author.
E-mail address: Dominique.delbeke@vanderbilt.edu (D. Delbeke).

PET Clin 3 (2008) 155–167
doi:10.1016/j.cpet.2008.08.008

Transabdominal US is well established as a valuable screening technique that is inexpensive, portable, and sensitive for evaluation of the pancreas, bile duct dilatation, and detection of hepatic lesions as small as 1 cm. It can also provide guidance for biopsy and drainage procedures. Its limitations include poor sensitivity (50%) for detection of small hepatic lesions and regional lymphadenopathy compared with CT and MR imaging.

Endoscopic ultrasound (EUS) is sensitive for the detection choledocolithiasis and pancreatic masses. However, it is highly operator-dependent and requires sedation.

CT is superior to US not only for detection of a pancreatic mass but also for assessment of vascular involvement and invasion of adjacent organs.

For hepatic imaging, CT and MR imaging are based on the dual perfusion of the liver: 80% of the blood flow to normal hepatic parenchyma is derived from the portal vein, whereas nearly all of the blood flow to hepatic neoplasms is derived from the hepatic artery. Therefore some lesions are better seen at different time after intravenous contrast injection. Typically, hypervascular tumors and metastases (hepatocellular carcinoma = HCC, metastases of carcinoid carcinoma, islet cell tumor, malignant pheochromocytoma, renal cell carcinoma, sarcoma, melanoma, and breast carcinoma) may be best seen during the arterial phase of enhancement, or before contrast is administered; whereas hypovascular metastases (colorectal carcinoma, and most metastases of other primaries) are best seen during the portal venous phase of enhancement.[3]

MR imaging is certainly as sensitive as CT for detection of focal hepatic lesions. A multitude of pulse sequences have been developed to characterize lesions. Gadolinium chelate contrast agents are used like the intravenous CT contrast agents, rapidly leaving the vascular space and reaching equilibrium throughout the extracellular fluid compartment after about 3 minutes.[4] Another contrast agent available for MR imaging of the liver is superparamagnetic iron oxide particles (SPIO), a marker of the reticuloendothelial cells (hepatic Kupffer cells). Most malignant tumors do not contain Kupffer cells and have a different T2 signal than normal hepatic parenchyma.

MR cholangiopancreatography (MRCP) permits visualization of the biliary tree noninvasively without the administration of contrast agents.[5] Using a heavily T2-weighted pulse sequence, solid organs and moving fluid have a low signal, whereas relatively stagnant fluid (such as bile) has a high signal intensity, resulting in the biliary tract appearing as a bright well-defined structure. Although MRCP does not provide the resolution of percutaneous transhepatic cholangiography (PTC) or endoscopic retrograde cholangiopancreatography (ERCP), it is able to clearly demonstrate intraluminal filling defects and luminal narrowing. MRCP provides invaluable information in both benign and malignant biliary tract disease.

Cholangiopancreatography via PTC or ERCP is an invasive technique but remains the procedure of choice for high-resolution assessment of the biliary tree anatomy. ERCP is performed by endoscopic cannulation of anatomic tracts and is therefore less invasive than PTC, which requires passage of a needle through the hepatic parenchyma. Contrast material is then injected directly into the biliary tree. Both techniques offer the advantage of allowing interventional procedures such as stent placement in the same setting as the imaging procedure. PTC demonstrates the intrahepatic ducts better than ERCP, which better depicts the extrahepatic ducts.

POSITRON EMISSION TOMOGRAPHY
18F-Fluorodeoxyglucose

Although variations in uptake are known to exist among tumor types, elevated uptake of ^{18}F-fluorodeoxyglucose (FDG) has been demonstrated in most primary malignant tumors.[6] This is because of the expression of increased numbers of glucose transporter proteins and increased intracellular enzyme levels of hexokinase and phosphofructokinase, among others, which promote glycolysis.[7–10] Pancreatic carcinoma does overexpress Glut-1.[11,12] Therefore, FDG PET imaging can be used to exploit the metabolic differences between benign and malignant cells for imaging purposes.[13,14]

Improvements in the distribution of FDG by commercial companies and the widespread oncologic applications including differentiation of benign from malignant lesions, staging malignant lesions, detection of malignant recurrence, and monitoring therapy have contributed to the establishment of the PET technology in many medical centers in the United States and Europe and progressively throughout the world. Because of the limitations of FDG related to variations of physiologic uptake and overlap of uptake between inflammatory and malignant lesions, other PET radiopharmaceuticals have been investigated for clinical use.

Instrumentation for Molecular Imaging with PET

The clinical utility of FDG imaging was first established using dedicated PET tomographs equipped with multiple rings of bismuth germanate oxide

(BGO) detectors, but a spectrum of equipment is now available for positron imaging including gamma camera-based PET at the low end of the spectrum and dedicated PET tomographs equipped with newer detector materials. The advantages and limitations of each of these systems is beyond the scope of this review.[15]

Although numerous studies have shown that the sensitivity and specificity of FDG imaging is superior to that of CT in many clinical settings, the inability of FDG imaging to provide accurate anatomic localization remains a significant impairment in maximizing its clinical utility. Because FDG is a tracer of glucose metabolism, its distribution is not limited to malignant tissue. To avoid misinterpretations, the interpreter must be familiar with the normal pattern and physiologic variations of FDG distribution and with clinical data relevant to the patient.[16,17] It is also important to standardize the environment of the patient during the uptake period so as to limit physiologic variations of FDG uptake.

The limitations of anatomic imaging with CT and MR imaging are related to size criteria for differentiation of benign from malignant lymph nodes, difficulty differentiating post-therapy changes from tumor recurrence, and difficulty differentiating non-opacified loops of bowel from metastases in the abdomen and pelvis.

Close correlation of FDG studies with conventional CT scans helps to minimize these difficulties. Interpretation has been traditionally accomplished by visually correlating FDG and CT images. In 2000, integrated PET/CT imaging systems became available commercially allowing optimal co-registration of images and became rapidly the standard of care.[18] Integrated SPECT/CT systems are also available and are becoming the standard of care when anatomic localization of SPECT anomalies is critical.

The CT portion of the study is most commonly acquired with low-mAs to reduce the radiation dose to the patient, although it can be acquired with diagnostic CT protocols. The reduced-dose CT is used for attenuation correction and anatomic localization with the help of the fusion of anatomic and molecular images. The incremental value of integrated PET/CT images compared with PET alone, or PET correlated with a CT obtained at a different time conclude the following: (1) improvement of lesion detection on both CT and FDG PET images, (2) improvement of the localization of foci of FDG uptake resulting in better differentiation of physiologic from pathologic uptake, and (3) precise localization of the malignant foci, for example in the skeleton versus soft tissue, or liver versus adjacent bowel or node. PET/CT

fusion images affect the clinical management by guiding further procedures, excluding the need of further procedures, and changing both inter- and intramodality therapy.[19] For example, precise localization of metastatic lymph nodes could result in a less invasive and more efficient surgical procedure. PET/CT fusion images have the potential to provide important information to guide the biopsy of a mass to more metabolically active regions of the tumor and to provide better maps than CT alone to modulate field and dose of radiation therapy.[20]

Integrated PET/CT and SPECT/CT imaging with integrated systems may be especially important in the abdomen and pelvis owing to the paucity of anatomic landmarks on functional imaging studies.[21] For example, FDG PET images alone may be difficult to interpret owing to the absence of anatomic landmarks (other than the liver, kidneys, and bladder); the presence of nonspecific uptake in the stomach, small bowel, and colon; and ureteral activity of FDG. Images of the abdomen and pelvis should be obtained with the arms elevated, whenever possible, to avoid artifacts due to motion and to beam hardening. A review of PET/CT for gastrointestinal tumors has been published.[22]

Summary

In summary, MDCT and EUS with FNA are the standard of care for evaluation of pancreatic cancer and detection of hepatic lesions, whereas US, MR imaging, MRCP, ERCP/PTC provide complementary techniques for further characterization of lesions in specific circumstances.

PET AND PET/CT FOR THE EVALUATION OF PANCREATIC CARCINOMA

The difficulty in correctly determining a preoperative diagnosis of pancreatic carcinoma is associated with two types of adverse outcomes. First, less aggressive surgeons may abort attempted resection because of a lack of tissue diagnosis. This is borne out by the significant rate of "reoperative" pancreaticoduodenectomy performed at major referral centers.[23–25] In a review of the M.D. Anderson Cancer Center involving 29 patients undergoing successful pancreaticoduodenectomy after failure to resect at the time of initial laparotomy, 31% did not undergo resection at the time of the initial procedure because of the lack of tissue confirmation of malignancy.[25] A second type of adverse outcome generated by failure to obtain a preoperative diagnosis occurs when more aggressive surgeons inadvertently resect benign disease. This is particularly notable in those patients who present with suspected malignancy without an associated mass on CT scan, occurring in up to 55% of patients.[26]

Preoperative Diagnosis of Pancreatic Carcinoma

Anatomic imaging modalities

The reported diagnostic accuracy of CT for detection of pancreatic cancer is in the 85% to 95% range.[27,28] The sensitivity and positive predictive value of dual-phase CT protocols for detection of pancreatic tumors are 97% and 92% respectively. Interpretation of the CT scan is sometimes difficult in the setting of mass-forming pancreatitis or other questionable findings, such as enlargement of the pancreatic head without definite signs of malignancy.[29,30] The diagnostic performance of MR imaging remains similar to that of CT. Even with the latest technology improvements, MR imaging demonstrates sensitivity of 86% and specificity of 89% for detection of pancreatic tumors.[31]

In a study of 80 patients with cancer, the sensitivity of EUS (98%) for detecting a pancreatic mass was greater than that of CT (86%).[28] In addition, EUS offers the possibility of tissue diagnosis with ultrasound-guided fine needle biopsy (FNA) with reported diagnostic yield of 68% and diagnostic accuracy of 74%.[32] The reported overall diagnostic rate, sensitivity, and negative predictive value of FNA biopsies guided using CT (98%, 95%, and 60%, respectively) are not significantly different from those guided using EUS (88.9%, 85%, and 57.%, respectively).[33]

The accuracy of ERCP is 80% to 90% for differentiation of benign from malignant pancreatic processes, including differentiation of tumor from chronic pancreatitis, because of the high degree of resolution of ductal structures that ERCP provides. The limitations of ERCP include false negatives when the tumor does not originate from the main duct, a 10% technical failure rate, and up to 8% morbidity (primarily iatrogenic pancreatitis). Principal advantages of ERCP include the ability to perform FNA biopsy and other interventional procedures (eg, sphincterotomy or stent placement). Although FNA biopsy may provide a tissue diagnosis, this technique suffers from significant sampling error.[34,35]

[18]F-fluorodeoxyglucose PET/CT for the preoperative diagnosis of pancreatic carcinoma

PET has a role in establishing the diagnosis of pancreatic carcinoma when the CT is nondiagnostic, when the biopsy is equivocal or nondiagnostic, when there is concurrent chronic pancreatitis, and for cystic lesions of the pancreas, even with the limitations of FDG PET imaging discussed in the section on limitations.

The summary of the literature published in 2001 reported average sensitivity and specificity of 94% and 90%, respectively.[6] All studies included have reported relatively high rates of sensitivity (85% to 100%), specificity (67% to 99%), and accuracy (85% to 93%) for ^{18}F-FDG PET imaging in the differentiation of benign from malignant pancreatic masses, and most suggest improved accuracy compared with CT. These results are similar to the findings in the series of Rose and colleagues[36] with a sensitivity of 92% and specificity of 85% for FDG PET compared with 65% and 62% respectively for CT imaging. FDG PET was particularly helpful in patients without a definite mass on CT and with nondiagnostic FNA. A recent review by Pakzad and colleagues[37] suggested that the overall sensitivity of FDG PET for detection of pancreatic carcinoma varies between 90% and 95% and specificity from 82% to 100%.

The performance of FDG PET was compared with CT and EUS for the diagnosis and staging of pancreatic cancer in 35 patients.[38] For the diagnosis, the sensitivity of EUS was 93%, compared with 87% for FDG PET and 53% for CT. EUS-guided FNA allowed tissue diagnosis in 67% of the patients.

FDG PET is more accurate than conventional imaging techniques (CT and MR) for differentiating benign from malignant cystic lesions of the pancreas and intraductal papillary mucinous tumors (IPMT). In a prospective study of 50 patients with suspected cystic pancreatic tumors, the sensitivity, specificity, positive and negative predictive value, and accuracy of FDG PET for detection of malignant tumors were 94%, 94%, 89%, 97%, and 94% compared with 65%, 88%, 73%, 83%, and 80% for CT.[39] In a series of 64 patients with suspected IPMT, the sensitivity of FDG PET was 80% (4/5) for carcinoma in situ and 95% (20/21) for invasive carcinoma, both superior to CT or MRCP, which were strongly suggestive of invasive carcinoma in only 62% of patients who had invasive carcinoma.[40] FDG uptake was absent in all adenomas (n = 13) and 87% (7/8) of borderline IPMNs. A positive FDG PET influenced the management of 10 patients with malignant IPMNs.

As for other malignancies, studies on a small number of patients suggest that the degree of FDG uptake in pancreatic malignancies correlates with the prognosis. Nakata and colleagues[41] noted an inverse correlation between standard uptake value (SUV) and survival in 14 patients with pancreatic adenocarcinoma. Patients with an SUV greater than 3.0 had a mean survival of 5 months compared with 14 months in those with an SUV less than 3.0. Zimny and colleagues[42] performed a multivariate analysis on 52 patients, including

SUV and accepted prognostic factors, to determine the prognostic value of FDG PET. The median survival of 26 patients with SUV greater than 6.1 was 5 months compared with 9 months for 26 patients with SUV less than 6.1. The multivariate analysis revealed that SUV and Ca 19-9 were independent factors for prognosis. Another study of 118 patients demonstrated that survival was significantly influenced by tumor stage, tumor grade, and SUV.[43]

Together, these series support the conclusion that FDG PET imaging may represent a useful adjunctive study in the evaluation of patients with suspected pancreatic cancer, especially when CT imaging results are inconclusive and/or FNA is nondiagnostic or there are cystic components.

Other PET Tracers for Diagnosis of Pancreatic Carcinoma

A pilot study of five patients compared ^{18}F-fluoro-L-thymidine (FLT) and FDG for detection of primary pancreatic adenocarcinoma, ^{18}F-FLT PET/CT scanning showed poor lesion detectability and relatively low levels of radiotracer uptake in the primary tumor compared with FDG.[44]

^{11}C-acetate does accumulate physiologically in the pancreas, allows rapid metabolic imaging using PET, and may be a useful metabolic probe for the study of pancreatic physiology and disease. However, adenocarcinoma of the pancreas demonstrated no significant uptake of ^{11}C-acetate.[45]

Staging of Pancreatic Carcinoma

In the TNM staging system for pancreatic cancer, Stage I disease is confined to the pancreas. Stage II disease is characterized by extrapancreatic extension (T stage), Stage III by lymph node involvement (N stage), and Stage IV by distant metastases (M stage) (**Tables 1** and **2**).

T staging can be evaluated only with anatomic imaging modalities, which demonstrate best the relationship between the tumor, adjacent organs, and vascular structures. Functional imaging modalities can obviously not replace anatomic imaging in the assessment of local tumor resectability. Sixty percent of patients presenting with pancreatic adenocarcinoma have advanced disease. Detection of nodal and peritoneal disease remains a challenge with all imaging modalities.

Conventional Imaging Modalities for Staging Pancreatic Carcinoma

The negative predictive value of CT for resectability is in the 85% to 95% range.[27,28] In a study using helical CT, CT had an accuracy of 91%, negative predictive value of 79%, and sensitivity of 91% for prediction of nonresectability. Helical CT allowed detection of vascular invasion in 88%, nodal involvement in 54%, and hepatic metastases in 75% of the cases.[46] Small hepatic and peritoneal metastases are difficult to detect on CT.[47] The evolution of CT technology has significantly improved the assessment of vascular involvement and invasion of adjacent organs with a negative predictive value of 100% for detection of vascular invasion and 87% for overall resectability.[27]

Compared with MDCT, EUS is superior for tumor detection and staging but similar for nodal staging and resectability of preoperatively suspected nonmetastatic pancreatic cancer.[28] In this study, the tumor staging accuracy was 67% for EUS compared with 41% for CT. The accuracy for nodal staging was 44% for EUS and 47% for CT. Of the 25 resectable pancreatic tumors in patients recommended for surgery, EUS and CT correctly identified 88% and 92%, respectively, as resectable. Of the 28 unresectable pancreatic tumors in patients recommended for surgery, EUS and CT correctly identified 68% and 64%, respectively, as unresectable.

In the study comparing the performance of FDG PET to CT and EUS for the diagnosis and staging of pancreatic cancer, EUS was more sensitive than CT for detecting vascular invasion of the portal and superior mesenteric veins.[38]

However, since many pancreatic cancers recur, including locally, the true definition of "resectability" probably shows somewhat limited good performance.

^{18}F-Fluorodeoxyglucose PET for Staging of Pancreatic Carcinoma

As for many other tumors, for T staging, there is no role for FDG PET; FDG imaging is not superior to contrast-enhanced MDCT for N staging, but it is more accurate than MDCT for M staging.[48]

For N staging, both CT and FDG PET are poor for detection of regional lymph node involvement with a reported sensitivity and specificity for FDG PET of 49% and 63%, respectively.[49]

FDG PET is most helpful and superior to CT for detection of distant unsuspected metastases and can often clarify the nature of equivocal CT lesions. For example, in a study by Delbeke and colleagues[48] metastases were diagnosed both on CT and on PET in 10 of 21 patients with stage IV disease, but PET demonstrated hepatic metastases not identified or equivocal on CT and/or distant metastases unsuspected clinically in seven additional patients (33%). In four patients (19%), neither CT nor PET imaging showed evidence of metastases,

Table 1
TNM classification for the staging of pancreatic cancer[71]

T (Tumor)	
TX	Primary tumor cannot be assessed.
T0	No evidence of primary tumor
Tis	Carcinoma in situ
T1	Tumor is ≤2 cm in greatest dimension and confined to pancreas.
T2	Tumor is >2 cm and confined to pancreas.
T3	Tumor extends beyond pancreas but does not involve celiac axis or superior mesenteric artery.
T4	Primary tumor involves either celiac axis or superior mesenteric artery.
N (Nodal involvement)	
NX	Regional lymph nodes cannot be assessed.
N0	No regional lymph node metastasis.
N1	Regional lymph node metastasis.
M (Metastases)	
MX	Distant metastasis cannot be assessed.
M0	No distant metastases.
M1	Distant metastasis.

Table 2
TNM stage grouping of pancreatic cancer

Stage	TNM Levels	Description
IA	T1 N0 M0	Resectable
IB	T2 N0 M0	
IIA	T3 N0M0	Typically resectable
IIB	T1-3 N1 M0	
III	T4 any N M0	Unresectable
IV	Any T any N M1	Unresectable

compared the performance of noninvasive imaging methods (US, CT, MR imaging, and FDG PET) in a mixed population of patients with colorectal, gastric, and esophageal cancers. At an equivalent specificity of 85%, FDG PET had the highest sensitivity of 90% compared with 76% for MR imaging, 72% for CT, and 55% for US for detection of hepatic metastases on a patient-based analysis.[50] A subsequent meta-analysis in 2005, including studies of MR imaging with gadolinium and superparamagnetic iron oxide particle (SPIO) enhancement, came to similar conclusions for patient-based analysis.[51] For a lesion-based analysis, FDG PET had the highest sensitivity of 76% compared with 66% for unenhanced MR imaging and 64% for CT. Both gadolinium- and SPIO-enhanced MR imaging were superior to nonenhanced MR imaging. SPIO MR imaging was the most sensitive technique with a sensitivity of 90% for detection of lesions greater than 1 cm, compared with 76% for FDG PET. In patients with colorectal cancer, FDG PET sensitivity for detection of hepatic metastases was compared with that of multiphase CT using intraoperative ultrasound as reference standard for lesions of different sizes.[52] The overall sensitivity was similar for PET (71%) and CT (72%); both PET and CT missed approximately 30% of smaller lesions resulting in a change of management in 7% of patients. There is one study comparing mangafodipir-trisodium–enhanced hepatic MR imaging with FDG PET for detection of hepatic metastases in patients with colorectal and pancreatic cancer.[53] Based on a per-patient analysis, MR imaging and FDG PET showed sensitivities of 97% and 93%, positive predictive values of 100% and 90%, and accuracies of 97% and 85%, respectively. According to a per-lesion analysis, MR imaging and FDG PET showed sensitivities of 81% and 67%, positive predictive values of 90% and 81%, and accuracies of 75% and 64%, respectively. FDG PET provided additional information about extrahepatic disease and was useful in initial staging. However, significantly more and smaller (subcentimeter)

but surgical exploration revealed carcinomatosis in three and a small hepatic metastasis in one patient. In the study of Mertz and colleagues,[38] FDG PET detected distant metastases in seven of nine proven metastases, four of which were missed by CT. An example of detection of distant metastasis with FDG PET/CT in a patient referred for initial staging is illustrated in **Fig. 1**.

A review by Pakzad and colleagues[37] suggested that the sensitivity of FDG PET for overall staging varies from 61% to 100% and specificity from 67% to 100%, not as good as for detection of the primary tumor.

Regarding detection of hepatic metastases, most studies comparing imaging studies have been performed in a mixed population of patients or patients with colorectal cancer metastatic to the liver. For example, a meta-analysis in 2002

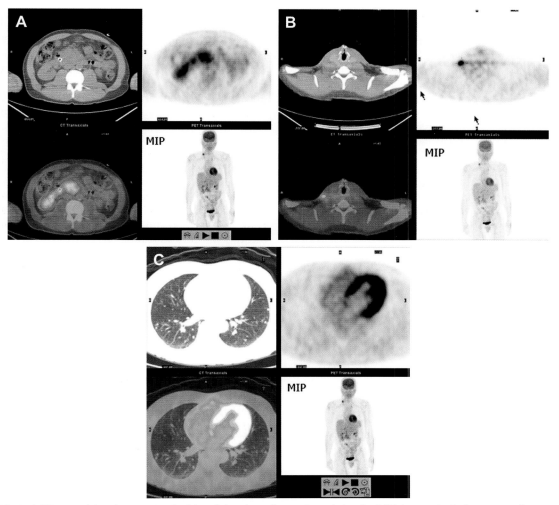

Fig.1. A 53-year-old male presented with painless jaundice and an abdominal CT demonstrated a pancreatic mass and pulmonary nodules at the lung bases. A fine needle aspiration of the pancreatic lesion demonstrated adenocarcinoma. The patient was referred to FDG PET/CT for initial staging. The fasting serum glucose was elevated to 154 mg/dL at the time of FDG administration. FDG PET maximum intensity projection (MIP) image demonstrates: **(1)** global decreased uptake in the brain most likely related to mild hyperglycemia or concurrent sedative medications, **(2)** focal FDG uptake in the right supraclavicular region, and **(3)** moderate FDG uptake in the region of the pancreatic head. Transaxial CT, FDG PET, and PET/CT fusion images demonstrate a large focus of moderate FDG uptake corresponding to the mass in the pancreatic head (*A*), intense uptake in a 1.2-cm supraclavicular lymph node (*B*) and innumerable small subcentimeter pulmonary nodules on CT, below PET resolution (*C*) consistent with a pancreatic primary adenocarcinoma with right supraclavicular lymph node, and pulmonary metastases. This case illustrates both detection of unsuspected metastases in the supraclavicular region with PET and pulmonary metastases on the CT portion of PET. Although the subcentimeter pulmonary lesions could not be definitively shown to be FDG-avid, the detection of an FDG-avid supraclavicular nodal metastasis is readily amenable to FNA biopsy, thus confirming stage IV disease.

hepatic metastases were detected on MR imaging than on FDG PET.

¹⁸F-Fluorodeoxyglucose PET/CT for Staging Pancreatic Carcinoma

The accuracy FDG PET/CT and impact on the management was reviewed in a series of 59 patients with suspected pancreatic cancer.[54] The accuracy of PET/CT for detection of pancreatic cancer was similar to previous studies using PET alone. Additional distant metastases were detected in five and synchronous rectal cancer in two patients. PET/CT findings changed the management in 16% of patients with pancreatic cancer deemed resectable after routine staging and was cost-saving.

In a study of 46 patients referred for staging or restaging pancreatic carcinoma, the fused PET/CT has a slightly higher sensitivity and accuracy rate for diagnosis and loco-regional staging of primary pancreatic lesions compared with CT alone. The accuracy of PET/CT (91%) for diagnosis of primary pancreatic lesions was marginally higher compared with CT (88%) and PET alone (82%). For loco-regional staging, PET/CT has a higher accuracy rate (85%) than PET alone (79%) but is similar to that of CT (84%). When used for restaging, sensitivity (90%) and accuracy (92%) were highest for PET and PET/CT compared with CT alone, which had a lower sensitivity (80%).[55]

A study of 82 patients demonstrated that the addition of PET/CT to standard CT of the abdomen and pelvis increased sensitivity (87%) for detection of metastatic disease in the initial work-up of patients with potentially resectable pancreatic neoplasms. The sensitivity and specificity of PET/CT in diagnosing pancreatic cancer were 89% and 88%, respectively. Sensitivity of detecting metastatic disease for PET/CT alone, standard CT alone, and the combination of PET/CT and CT were 61%, 57%, and 87%, respectively. Findings on PET/CT influenced the clinical management in seven patients (11%), two with a supra-clavicular lymph node, two with occult hepatic lesions, two with peritoneal implants, and one with peri-esophageal lymph nodes.[56]

[18]F-Fluorodeoxyglucose PET in the Post-Therapy Setting

The value of FDG PET for monitoring therapy and detection of recurrence of pancreatic carcinoma has been reported in several studies. FDG PET may be particularly useful for evaluation of an indistinct abnormality in the resection bed seen on CT, which is difficult to differentiate from surgical- or radiation-induced fibrosis, for evaluation of newly seen hepatic lesions that may be too small to biopsy, and for restaging of patients with rising serum tumor marker levels and a negative conventional work-up. A study of 31 patients with suspected recurrent pancreatic carcinoma compared the performance of FDG PET to CT or MR imaging. FDG PET detected 96% (22/23) of the patients with recurrence compared with 39% (9/23) for CT or MR imaging. MR imaging or CT detected more hepatic metastases than FDG PET but FDG PET detected 100% (7/7) of the extrahepatic abdominal recurrences and two extra-abdominal recurrences, whereas none were detected by CT or MR imaging.[57] An

example of an extra-abdominal recurrence detected on PET/CT imaging is illustrated in **Fig. 2**.

Preliminary data also suggest that FDG PET imaging is useful for the assessment of tumor response to neoadjuvant therapy. In the study of Rose and colleagues,[36] nine patients had pre- and posttreatment FDG-PET to assess the response to neoadjuvant chemo-radiation in patients with potentially resectable pancreatic cancer. Four patients had evidence of tumor response by PET (reduction in tumor FDG uptake of $\geq 50\%$) without evidence of change in size on CT, and all four patients went on to successful resection, all with histologic evidence of 20% to 80% tumor necrosis. Three patients showed stable disease, and two showed tumor progression. Among the two patients with progressive disease documented by FDG-PET, one showed tumor progression on CT and the other demonstrated stable disease. Among the five patients who showed no response by FDG-PET, the disease could subsequently be resected in only two, and only one patient who underwent resection showed evidence of chemo-radiation effect in the resected specimen.

Impact of ^{18}F-Fluorodeoxyglucose PET/CT on the Management of Patients with Pancreatic Carcinoma

A summary of the FDG PET literature published in 2001 reported a change in management induced by FDG PET in 36% of patients. Delbeke and colleagues[48] reported a series of 65 patients in whom the addition of FDG-PET imaging to CT altered the surgical management in 41% of the patients, either by detection of CT-occult pancreatic carcinoma (27%) or by identification of unsuspected distant metastases (14%). The addition of FDG-PET imaging to CT was also helpful in the verification of the benign nature of equivocal findings seen on CT. In this regard, FDG-PET allows selection of the optimal surgical approach to patients with pancreatic carcinoma.

Kalady and colleagues[58] reviewed the performance of FDG PET in 54 patients with suspected periampullary malignancy. Despite high sensitivity (88%) and specificity (86%) of FDG-PET in diagnosing periampullary malignancy compared with CT (sensitivity 90%, specificity 62%), FDG-PET did not change clinical management in the vast majority of patients previously evaluated by CT. In addition, FDG-PET missed more than 10% of periampullary malignancies and did not provide the anatomic detail necessary to define resectability.

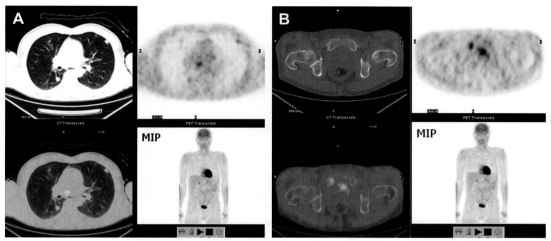

Fig. 2. A 50-year-old diabetic male with a history of pancreatic carcinoma and prior Whipple resection presented with new pulmonary nodules on CT. A fine needle aspiration was nondiagnostic. The patient was referred to FDG PET/CT for restaging. The fasting serum glucose level was elevated to 174 mg/dL at the time of FDG administration. FDG PET MIP image demonstrated diffuse muscular uptake and globally decreased uptake in the brain most likely related to hyperglycemia, thus decreasing the sensitivity for detection of FDG-avid lesions. However, there are foci of mild uptake over the lung fields and a focus of FDG uptake in the right lower pelvis below the bladder. Transaxial views through the foci of uptake in the lungs demonstrated corresponding pulmonary nodules with the ones above PET resolution being FDG-avid (A). The focus of FDG uptake in the pelvis corresponds to a lytic lesion in the right pubic ramus consistent with a skeletal metastasis (B). Therefore, despite the limitations of diabetic hyperglycemia and the accompanying diminished sensitivity for detection of metastases, FDG PET/CT was able to confirm that the larger lung nodules were FDG-avid and likely metastatic. The incidental detection of an FDG-avid skeletal metastasis confirmed stage IV disease.

In 2000, the European consensus conference designated FDG PET as an established indication for differentiation of benign and malignant pancreatic masses.[59] However, the performance of FDG PET or PET/CT for the evaluation of pancreatic carcinoma is still not covered by the Centers for Medicare and Medicaid Services (CMS) in the United States in 2008.

Limitations of ^{18}F-Fluorodeoxyglucose Imaging

Scintigraphic tumor detectability depends on both the size of the lesion and the degree of uptake, as well as surrounding background uptake and intrinsic resolution of the imaging system. Small lesions may yield false-negative results because of partial volume averaging, leading to underestimation of the uptake in lesions less than twice the resolution of the imaging system. For example, mucinous tumors, small ampullary carcinoma, military spread of tumor, and necrotic lesions with a thin viable rim can be false-negative. The sensitivity of FDG PET for detection of mucinous adenocarcinoma is lower than for nonmucinous adenocarcinoma (41% to 58% versus 92%), probably because of the relative hypocellularity of these tumors.[60] The detection rate for ampullary carcinoma with FDG imaging is only 70% to 80%, probably because of their smaller size at the time of clinical presentation (**Fig. 3**A).[58] In addition, such lesions can be located to adjacent FDG-avid bowel, thus lowering tumor/background ratios.

Hyperglycemia decreases tumor uptake because of competitive inhibition. The high incidence of glucose intolerance and diabetes exhibited by patients with pancreatic pathology represents a potential limitation of this modality in the diagnosis of pancreatic cancer. Low SUV values and false-negative FDG-PET scans have been noted in hyperglycemic patients compared with euglycemic patients.[61–63] Some investigators have suggested various methods to correct or compensate the measured SUV based on serum glucose levels at the time of the radiopharmaceutical injection.[49,63–65] For example, in a study of 106 patients with a prevalence of disease of 70%, Zimny and colleagues[62] found that FDG PET had a sensitivity of 98% in a subgroup of euglycemic patients compared with 63% in a subgroup of hyperglycemic patients. Conversely, some investigators[66,67] have noted no variation in the accuracy of FDG PET based on serum glucose levels.

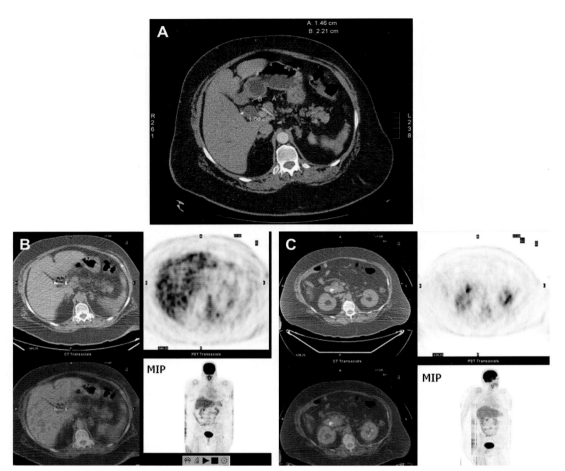

Fig. 3. A 62-year-old female presented with jaundice. CT demonstrated extrahepatic biliary obstruction with the common bile duct measuring 1.8 cm and a 1.5-cm low attenuation lesion in the periampullary/pancreatic head region (*A*). ERCP-directed biopsy revealed invasive adenocarcinoma. A biliary stent was placed and the patient was referred to FDG PET/CT imaging for initial staging. Transaxial views through the lesion seen on CT and ERCP shows no significant FDG uptake (*B*). Ampullary carcinoma can be false-negative on FDG PET owing to their small size and possible mucinous component. There is a focus of FDG uptake corresponding to the stent in the pancreatic duct (*C*). This could be related to inflammatory changes induced by placement of the stent 2 weeks earlier. An exploratory laparotomy demonstrated a 1.5-cm periampullary adenocarcinoma extending into the adjacent pancreas. Increased FDG uptake along the course of a biliary stent should not be confused with a malignant process. Although FDG PET maybe useful in the detection of loco-regional or distant metastases, in patients with suspected periampullary carcinoma, a negative FDG PET examination cannot exclude the presence of a primary periampullary neoplasm.

In view of the known high uptake of FDG by activated macrophages, neutrophils, fibroblasts, and granulation tissue, it is not surprising that inflammatory tissue exhibits increased FDG activity. Mild to moderate FDG activity seen early after radiation therapy, along recent incisions, infected incisions, biopsy sites, drainage tubing, and catheters, as well as colostomy sites can lead to errors in interpretation if the history is not known. Some inflammatory lesions, especially granulomatous ones, may be markedly FDG-avid and can be mistaken for malignancies; this includes inflammatory bowel disease, abscesses, acute cholangitis, acute cholecystitis and acute pancreatitis, and chronic active pancreatitis with or without abscess formation.[68] Nonetheless, FDG PET is able to detect pancreatic carcinoma in the setting of chronic pancreatitis with a sensitivity of 92% (24/26) and a negative predictive value of 87%.[69] False-positive studies are frequent in patients with elevated C-reactive protein (CRP) and/or acute pancreatitis, with a specificity as low as 50% when the CRP serum level is elevated compared with 86% when CRP level is normal.[62,63,66]

Therefore, correlation the FDG PET findings with a CRP level is recommended.

Other lesions with false-positive findings that have been reported include serous cystadenoma, retroperitoneal fibrosis, and inflammatory changes around stents (**Fig. 3**B). False-positive findings have been reported in the liver of patients with intrahepatic cholestasis with dilated bile ducts and from inflammatory granulomas.[70]

SUMMARY

FDG PET imaging is especially helpful for the preoperative diagnosis of pancreatic carcinoma in patients with suspected pancreatic cancer in whom CT fails to identify a discrete tumor mass or in whom FNAs are nondiagnostic. By providing preoperative documentation of pancreatic malignancy in these patients, laparotomy may be undertaken with a curative intent, and the risk of aborting resection because of diagnostic uncertainty is minimized. FDG PET imaging is also useful for M staging and restaging by detecting CT-occult metastatic disease, and allowing noncurative resection to be avoided altogether in this group of patients. As is true with other neoplasms, FDG PET can differentiate post-therapy changes from recurrence and holds promise for monitoring neoadjuvant chemoradiation therapy.

FDG PET is less useful in periampullary carcinoma and marginally helpful in staging except for M staging.

As for other malignancies, FDG PET imaging is complementary to morphologic imaging with CT; therefore, integrated PET/CT imaging provides optimal images for interpretation. The diagnostic implications of integrated PET/CT imaging include improved detection of lesions on both the CT and FDG PET images, better differentiation of physiologic from pathologic foci of metabolism, and better localization of the pathologic foci. This new powerful technology provides more accurate interpretation of both CT and FDG PET images and therefore more optimal patient care. PET/CT fusion images affect the clinical management by guiding further procedures (biopsy, surgery, radiation therapy), excluding the need for additional procedures, and changing both inter- and intramodality therapy.

REFERENCES

1. American Cancer Society. Cancer facts and figures 2007: year 2007 surveillance research from the American Cancer Society. Bethseda (MD): American Cancer Society; 2007.

2. Faria SC, Tamm EP, Loyer EM, et al. Diagnosis and staging of pancreatic tumors. Semin Roentgenol 2004;39(3):397–411.

3. Kemmerer SC, Mortele KJ, Ros PR. CT scan of the liver. Radiol Clin North Am 1998;36(2):247–60.

4. Siegelman ES, Outwater EK. MR imaging technique of the liver. Radiol Clin North Am 1998;36(2):263–84.

5. Fulcher AS, Turner MA, Capps GW. MR cholangiography: technical advances and clinical applications. Radiographics 1999;19(1):25–43.

6. Gambhir SS, Czernin J, Schwimmer J, et al. A tabulated summary of the FDG PET literature. J Nucl Med 2001;42(Suppl 1):1S–93S.

7. Warburg O. Versuche und uberledbeudem carcinomgewebe (methoden). Biochem Z 1923;142:317–33.

8. Flier JS, Mueckler MM, Usher P, et al. Elevated levels of glucose transport and transporter messenger RNA are induced by rats or src oncogenes. Science 1987;235:1492–5.

9. Monakhov NK, Neistadt EI, Shaylovskii MM, et al. Physiochemical properties and isoenzyme composition of hexokinase from normal and malignant human tissues. J Natl Cancer Inst 1978;61:27–34.

10. Knox WE, Jamdar SC, Davis PA. Hexokinase, differentiation, and growth rates of transplanted tumors. Cancer Res 1970;30:2240–4.

11. Higashi T, Tamaki N, Honda T, et al. Expression of glucose transporters in human pancreatic tumors compared with increased F-18 FDG accumulation in PET study. J Nucl Med 1997;38:1337–44.

12. Reske S, Grillenberger KG, Glatting G, et al. Overexpression of glucose transporter 1 and increased F-18 FDG uptake in pancreatic carcinoma. J Nucl Med 1997;38:1344–8.

13. Som P, Atkins HL, Bandoypadhayay D, et al. A fluorinated glucose analog, 2-fluoro-2-deoxy-2-D-glucose [18F]: nontoxic tracer for rapid tumor detection. J Nucl Med 1980;21:670–5.

14. Gallagher BM, Fowler JS, Gutterson NI, et al. Metabolic trapping as a principle of radiopharmaceutical design: some factors responsible for the biodistribution of [18F]2-deoxy-2-fluoro-D-glucose. J Nucl Med 1978;19:1154–61.

15. Townsend DW, Carney JPJ, Yap JT, et al. PET/CT today and tomorrow. J Nucl Med 2004;45(Suppl 1):4S–14S.

16. Cook GJR, Fogelman I, Maisey MN. Normal physiological and benign pathological variants of 18-fluoro-2-deoxyglucose positron emission tomography scanning: potential for error in interpretation. Semin Nucl Med 1996;26:308–14.

17. Engel H, Steinert H, Buck A, et al. Whole body PET: physiological and artifactual fluorodeoxyglucose accumulations. J Nucl Med 1996;37:441–6.

18. Townsend DW, Beyer T, Bloggett TM. PET/CT scanners: a hardware approach to image fusion. Semin Nucl Med 2003;33(3):193–204.

19. Czernin J. PET/CT: imaging structure and function. J Nucl Med 2004;45(Suppl 1):1S–103S.

20. Ciernik IF, Dizendorf E, Baumert BG, et al. Radiation treatment planning with integrated positron emission and computed tomography (PET/CT): a feasibility study. Int J Radiat Oncol Biol Phys 2003;57(3): 853–63.

21. Wahl RL. Why nearly all PET of abdominal and pelvic cancer will be performed as PET/CT. J Nucl Med 2004;45(Suppl 1):82S–95S.

22. Schoder H, Larson SM, Yeung WD. PET/CT in oncology: integration into clinical management of lymphoma, melanoma and gastrointestinal malignancies. J Nucl Med 2004;45(Suppl 1):72S–81S.

23. McGuire GE, Pitt HA, Lillemoe KD, et al. Reoperative surgery for periampullary adenocarcinoma. Arch Surg 1991;126:1205–12.

24. Tyler DS, Evans DB. Reoperative pancreaticoduodenectomy. Ann Surg 1994;219:211–21.

25. Robinson EK, Lee JE, Lowy AM, et al. Reoperative pancreaticoduodenectomy for periampullary carcinoma. Am J Surg 1996;172:432–8.

26. Thompson JS, Murayama KM, Edney JA, et al. Pancreaticoduodenectomy for suspected but unproven malignancy. Am J Surg 1994;169:571–5.

27. Vargas R, Nino-Murcia M, Trueblood W, et al. MDCT in pancreatic adenocarcinoma: prediction of vascular invasion and resectability using a multiphasic technique with curved planar reformations. AJR Am J Roentgenol 2004;182(2):419–25.

28. DeWitt J, Devereaux B, Chriswell M, et al. Comparison of endoscopic ultrasonography and multidetector computed tomography for detecting and staging pancreatic cancer. Ann Intern Med 2004;141(10): 753–63.

29. Johnson PT, Outwater EK. Pancreatic carcinoma versus chronic pancreatitis: dynamic MR imaging. Radiology 1999;212(1):213–8.

30. Lammer J, Herlinger H, Zalaudek G, et al. Pseudotumorous pancreatitis. Gastrointest Radiol 1995;10: 59–67.

31. Birchard KR, Semelka RC, Hyslop WB, et al. Evaluation of pancreatic cancer by MRI. Am J Roentgenol 2005;185:700–3.

32. Voss M, Hammel P, Molas G, et al. Value of endoscopic ultrasound guided fine needle aspiration biopsy in the diagnosis of solid pancreatic masses. Gut 2000;46(2):244–9.

33. Erturk SM, Mortele KJ, Tuncali K, et al. Fine-needle aspiration biopsy of solid pancreatic masses: comparison of CT and endoscopic sonography guidance. Am J Roentgenol 2006;187(6):1531–5.

34. Brandt KR, Charboneau JW, Stephens DH, et al. CT- and US-guided biopsy of the pancreas. Radiology 1993;187:99–104.

35. Chang KJ, Nguyen P, Erickson RA, et al. The clinical utility of endoscopic ultrasound-guided fine-needle aspiration in the diagnosis and staging of pancreatic carcinoma. Gastrointest Endosc 1997;45:387–93.

36. Rose DM, Delbeke D, Beauchamp RD, et al. 18Fluorodeoxyglucose - positron emission tomography (18FDG - PET) in the management of patients with suspected pancreatic cancer. Ann Surg 1998;229: 729–38.

37. Pakzad F, Groves AM, Ell PJ. The role of positron emission tomography in the management of pancreatic cancer. Semin Nucl Med 2006;36(3): 248–56.

38. Mertz HR, Sechopoulos P, Delbeke D, et al. EUS, PET, and CT scanning for evaluation of pancreatic adenocarcinoma. Gastrointest Endosc 2000;52(3): 367–71.

39. Sperti C, Pasquali C, Decet G, et al. F-18-fluorodeoxyglucose positron emission tomography in differentiating malignant from benign pancreatic cysts: a prospective study. J Gastrointest Surg 2005;(1):22–8 [discussion: 28–9].

40. Sperti C, Bissoli S, Pasquali C, et al. 18-Fluorodeoxyglucose positron emission tomography enhances computed tomography diagnosis of malignant intraductal papillary mucinous neoplasms of the pancreas. Ann Surg 2007;246(6):932–9.

41. Nakata B, Chung YS, Nishimura S, et al. 18F-fluorodeoxyglucose positron emission tomography and the prognosis of patients with pancreatic carcinoma. Cancer 1997;79:695–9.

42. Zimny M, Fass J, Bares R, et al. Fluorodeoxyglucose positron emission tomography and the prognosis of pancreatic carcinoma. Scand J Gastroenterol 2000; 35:883–8.

43. Sperti C, Pasquali C, Chierichetti F, et al. 18-Fluorodeoxyglucose positron emission tomography in predicting survival of patients with pancreatic carcinoma. J Gastrointest Surg 2003;7(8):953–9.

44. Quon A, Chang ST, Chin F, et al. Initial evaluation of 18F-fluorothymidine (FLT) PET/CT scanning for primary pancreatic cancer. Eur J Nucl Med Mol Imaging. 2008; 35(3):527–31. Epub 2007 Oct 25.

45. Shreve PD, Gross MD. Imaging of the pancreas and related diseases with PET carbon-11-acetate. J Nucl Med 1997;38(8):1305–10.

46. Diehl SJ, Lehman KJ, Sadick M, et al. Pancreatic cancer: value of dual-phase helical CT in assessing resectability. Radiology 1998;206:373–8.

47. Bluemke DA, Cameron IL, Hurban RH, et al. Potentially resectable pancreatic adenocarcinoma: spiral CT assessment with surgical and pathologic correlation. Radiology 1995;197:381–5.

48. Delbeke D, Rose M, Chapman WC, et al. Optimal interpretation of F-18FDG imaging of FDG PET in the diagnosis, staging and management of pancreatic carcinoma. J Nucl Med 1999;40:1784–92.

49. Diederichs CG, Staib L, Vogel J, et al. Values and limitations of FDG PET with preoperative evaluations

of patients with pancreatic masses. Pancreas 2000; 20:109–16.

50. Kinkel K, Lu Y, Both M, et al. Detection of hepatic metastases from cancers of the gastrointestinal tract by using noninvasive imaging methods (US, CT, MR imaging, PET): a meta-analysis. Radiology 2002; 224(3):748–56.

51. Bipat S, van Leeuwen MS, Comans EF, et al. Colorectal liver metastases: CT, MR imaging, and PET for diagnosis–meta-analysis. Radiology 2005; 237(1):123–31.

52. Wiering B, Ruers TJ, Krabbe PF, et al. Comparison of multiphase CT, FDG-PET and intra-operative ultrasound in patients with colorectal liver metastases selected for surgery. Ann Surg Oncol 2007;14(2):818–26.

53. Sahani DV, Kalva SP, Fischman AJ, et al. Detection of liver metastases from adenocarcinoma of the colon and pancreas: comparison of mangafodipir trisodium-enhanced liver MRI and whole-body FDG PET. AJR Am J Roentgenol 2005;185(1):239–46.

54. Heinrich S, Goerres GW, Schäfer M, et al. Positron emission tomography/computed tomography influences on the management of resectable pancreatic cancer and its cost-effectiveness. Ann Surg 2005; 242(2):235–43.

55. Casneuf V, Delrue L, Kelles A, et al. Is combined 18F-fluorodeoxyglucose-positron emission tomography/computed tomography superior to positron emission tomography or computed tomography alone for diagnosis, staging and restaging of pancreatic lesions? Acta Gastroenterol Belg 2007; 70(4):331–8.

56. Farma JM, Santillan AA, Melis M, et-al. PET/CT fusion scan enhances CT staging in patients with pancreatic neoplasms. Ann Surg Oncol 2008 [Epub ahead of print].

57. Ruf J, Lopez Hänninen E, Oettle H, et al. Detection of recurrent pancreatic cancer: comparison of FDG-PET with CT/MRI. Pancreatology 2005;5(2–3):266–72.

58. Kalady MF, Clary BM, Clark LA, et al. Clinical utility of positron emission tomography in the diagnosis and management of periampullary neoplasms. Ann Surg Oncol 2002;9(8):799–806.

59. Reske SN, Kotzerke J. FDG-PET for clinical use. Results of the 3rd German interdisciplinary consensus conference, "Onko-PET III," 21 July and 19 September 2000. Eur J Nucl Med 2001;28:1707–23.

60. Whiteford MH, Whiteford HM, Yee LF, et al. Usefulness of FDG-PET scan in the assessment of suspected metastatic or recurrent adenocarcinoma of the colon and rectum. Dis Colon Rectum 2000; 43(6):759–67 [discussion: 767–0].

61. Stollfuss JC, Glatting G, Friess H, et al. 2-(Fluorine-18)-fluoro-2-deoxy-D-glucose PET in detection of pancreactic cancer: value of quantitative image interpretation. Radiology 1995;195:339–44.

62. Zimny M, Bares R, Faß J, et al. Fluorine-18 fluorodeoxyglucose positron emission tomography in the differential diagnosis of pancreatic carcinoma: a report of 106 cases. Eur J Nucl Med 1997;24: 678–82.

63. Wahl RL, Henry CA, Ethrer SP. Serum glucose: effects on tumor and normal tissue accumulation of 2-[F-18]-fluoro-2-deoxy-D-glucose in rodents with mammary carcinoma. Radiology 1992;183:643–7.

64. Lindholm P, Minn H, Leskinen-Kallio S, et al. Influence of the blood glucose concentration on FDG uptake in cancer—a PET study. J Nucl Med 1993;34: 1–6.

65. Diederichs CG, Staib L, Glatting G, et al. FDG PET: elevated plasma glucose reduces both uptake and detection rate of pancreatic malignancies. J Nucl Med 1998;39:1030–3.

66. Ho CL, Dehdashti F, Griffeth LK, et al. FDG-PET evaluation of indeterminate pancreatic masses. J Comput Assist Tomogr 1996;20:363–9.

67. Friess H, Langhans J, Ebert M, et al. Diagnosis of pancreatic cancer by 2[F-18]-fluoro-2-deoxy-D-glucose positron emission tomography. Gut 1995;36: 771–7.

68. Shreve PD. Focal fluorine-18 fluorodeoxyglucose accumulation in inflammatory pancreatic disease. Eur J Nucl Med 1998;25:259–64.

69. van Kouwen M, Jansen JB, van Goor H, et al. FDG-PET is able to detect pancreatic carcinoma in chronic pancreatitis. Eur J Nucl Med Mol Imaging 2005;32(4):399–404.

70. Frolich A, Diederichs CG, Staib L, et al. Detection of liver metastases from pancreatic cancer using FDG PET. J Nucl Med 1999;40:250–5.

71. AJCC cancer staging manual. 6th edition. Springer; 2004. Available at: http://www.cancer.gov/cancertopics/pdq/treatment/pancreatic/healthprofessional. Accessed October 13, 2008.

Primary Cancer of the Liver and Biliary Duct

Jong Doo Lee, MD, PhD*, Won Jun Kang, MD, PhD, Mijin Yun, MD, PhD

KEYWORDS

- Hepatocellular carcinoma • Cholangiocarcinoma
- Positron emission tomography
- Fluorodeoxyglucose • Acetate

PRIMARY CANCER OF THE LIVER AND BILIARY DUCT

Hepatocellular Carcinoma

Hepatocellular carcinoma (HCC) is the most common primary hepatic malignancy, accounting for up to 85% to 90%, and the incidence of HCC is increasing worldwide.[1–3] Positron emission tomography (PET) using fluorine-18-fluorodeoxyglucose (F-18-FDG) is useful in staging, prediction of prognosis, evaluation of recurrence, and treatment response in HCCs; however; the high false-negative rate in detecting primary HCC (40%–50%) limits its use. With regard to histopathologic differentiation of HCC, the most consistent factor contributing to FDG uptake in tumors is different glucose metabolism.[4–9]

Recently, carbon-11 (C-11)-acetate has been shown to be useful in detecting those HCCs not seen on F-18-FDG PET studies.[10] Therefore, awareness of the pathophysiologic mechanisms underlying cancer energy metabolism, especially glucose and fatty acid metabolism in HCCs, will improve the diagnostic usefulness of PET or PET-CT.

Differences in glucose metabolism between normal hepatocytes and hepatocellular carcinomas

The liver is the major organ for the production of glucose, at a rate of 2.0 mg/kg/min, to maintain glucose homeostasis, which is balanced with glucose use.[11] In the postprandial state, dietary carbohydrates are absorbed in the small intestine. Glucose is transported into the enterocytes by sodium-dependent glucose transporter-1 (SGLT-1) using the electrochemical gradient of sodium, then released into the interstitial space by facilitated diffusion, by way of glucose transporter (GLUT) type 2 (GLUT-2) or other unknown mechanisms.[12] Glucose in the bloodstream is transported into the liver to replenish glycogen storage or for glycolysis for energy requirements. The transport of glucose into the liver is facilitated mainly by high Km and low-affinity GLUT-2, which is distributed on the microvilli of the sinusoidal plasma membrane. The level of GLUT-2 mRNA in periportal hepatocytes is higher than in perivenous hepatocytes, and GLUT-1 is mainly present in the perivenous hepatocytes.[13] Recently, GLUT-8 has also been shown to be expressed in the liver for glucose homeostasis.[14]

Glucose in the liver is used for energy production and for the synthesis of amino acids, fatty acids, or nucleotides, and is phosphorylated to glucose-6-phosphate (G6P) by glycolytic enzyme, hexokinase (HK) family (type I–IV) during first phase of glycolysis. HK I to III are about 100 kDa in size and are inhibited by G6P. However, HK IV, known as glucokinase, is a key enzyme in the liver and is approximately 50 kDa in size but is not significantly affected by physiologic concentration of G6P.[15,16] G6P is a central metabolite in the liver for the production of pyruvate to generate ATP, for the synthesis of glycogen, fatty acids, and nucleotides, and for gluconeogenesis by way of glucose-6-phosphatase (G6Pase).[11] Therefore, transcription of downstream glycolytic enzymes and their related molecules, such as pyruvate kinase, fatty acid synthase, G6Pase, and GLUT-2, is stimulated by enhanced glucose metabolism in the liver.[17–20]

In malignant tumor cells in the liver, liver-specific GLUT-2 and glycolytic enzyme glucokinase are

Division of Nuclear Medicine, Department of Diagnostic Radiology, Yonsei University College of Medicine, 250 Seongsan-ro, Seodaemun-gu, Seoul 120-752, South Korea
* Corresponding author.
E-mail address: jdlee@yuhs.ac (J.D. Lee).

PET Clin 3 (2008) 169–186
doi:10.1016/j.cpet.2008.08.005
1556-8598/08/$ – see front matter © 2008 Elsevier Inc. All rights reserved.

replaced by GLUT-1 and HK II or HK I,[21,22] respectively, to facilitate high rates of glucose catabolism. In the early 1930s, Otto Warburg, the German biochemist, showed that many tumor cells exhibit a high rate of glycolysis, and cancer cells can obtain approximately the same amount of energy from fermentation (lactic acid) as from mitochondrial respiration, even in the presence of oxygen (the "Warburg effect") (**Fig. 1**).[23,24] The Warburg effect has become a basic mechanism of F-18-FDG uptake on PET scan that enables proper diagnosis, prognostic stratification, monitoring of therapy response, and evaluation of recurrence in malignant tumors. Since the discovery of the Warburg effect, molecular studies have revealed multiple genetic alterations in glycolytic pathways in tumor cells. For example, a hypoxic condition in tumors induces a well-known transcription factor, hypoxia inducible factor-1 (HIF-1). It binds to the DNA sequence of promoters in many related genes, and the expression of glycolytic enzymes, including HK, pyruvate kinase M, and vascular endothelial growth factor, is increased.[25] In addition, isotype switching of key enzymes, such as phosphofructokinase[26] and pyruvate kinase,[27] accelerates cancer metabolism and tumor growth. Recently, it has been reported that isotype switching from type M1 isoform of pyruvate kinase to the embryonic type M2 isoform of pyruvate kinase plays a major role in lactate production (the Warburg effect) in tumor cells. Instead, adult-type M1 isoform reduces lactate production, which is a reversal of the Warburg effect.[27]

These metabolic alterations of glycolytic pathways with related gene regulations provide insights regarding the prognostic implications and histopathologic differentiation of tumors based on the F-18-FDG uptake patterns.

F-18-fluorodeoxyglucose uptake mechanisms in hepatocellular carcinomas

F-18-FDG uptake is increased in high-grade and poorly differentiated HCCs but it is minimally increased or almost identical to the surrounding normal hepatocyte uptake in low-grade HCCs (**Fig. 2**), which makes it difficult to detect low-grade HCCs using F-18-FDG PET alone. However, even well-differentiated HCC does not produce a photon defect or significantly lower uptake than surrounding normal parenchyma on F-18-FDG PET scan, as other benign lesions such as hepatic cysts do, which could aid in the differential diagnosis between HCCs and nonmalignant lesions (**Fig. 3**).

In terms of F-18-FDG uptake mechanisms in HCCs, molecular works using animal models or cell lines have demonstrated a large excess of GLUT activity over HK I or II activity.[28] On the other hand, studies on the immunohistochemical analysis of the GLUT-1 in HCCs showed low incidence of GLUT-1 expression even in high-grade HCCs, but increased HK II expression.[29–31] The variable expression patterns of GLUTs and HKs are not unusual in malignant tumors. Indeed, previous studies using human melanoma tissues also have demonstrated variation of expression of these molecules, a 22-fold variation of GLUT-1 and a 9-fold variation of HK expression, because of the heterogeneity of the biologic properties in the tumor cells.[32] Basically, the total amount of these proteins is not always coupled with their activity. In addition, F-18-FDG uptake appears to be more correlated with the FDG phosphorylating activity of the mitochondrial-bound HKs than GLUT-1.[33]

Another important factor affecting F-18-FDG uptake could be G6Pase activity, which releases glucose back to the bloodstream. These mechanisms affect the intracellular concentration of the transported F-18-FDG. In normal hepatocyte, G6Pase dephosphorylates G6P to glucose; then, intracytoplasmic glucose is released for homeostasis by using a facilitated diffusion mechanism by way of the GLUT-2 system on the sinusoidal membrane of hepatocytes[34] or an alternative

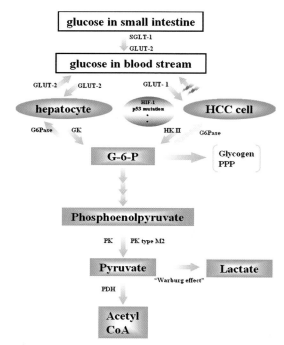

Fig. 1. Glycolytic pathway in normal hepatocytes and HCC cells. CoA, coenzyme A; GK, glucokinase; HIF, hypoxia inducible factor; p53, protein 53; PDH, pyruvate dehydrogenase; PK, pyruvate kinase; PPP, pentose phosphate pathway.

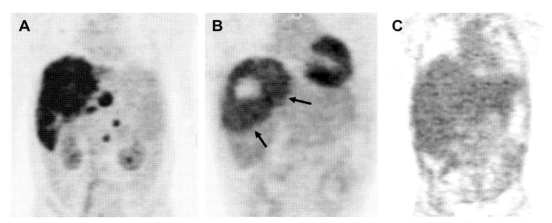

Fig. 2. Various F-18-FDG uptake patterns in HCCs. The F-18-FDG uptake pattern is well correlated with histopathologic grading in HCCs. (*A*) F-18-FDG uptake is intensely increased in high-grade HCC and (*B*) moderately increased in intermediate HCCs or mixed high- and low-grade HCC cells (*arrows*). (*C*) Uptake is not significantly increased in low-grade HCCs.

membrane trafficking mechanism. The presence of alternative membrane trafficking mechanisms has been demonstrated by Guillam and colleagues[35] in a GLUT-2 null mice model.

Previous study has suggested that low F-18-FDG uptake in low-grade HCCs could be due to high G6Pase but low HK activities;[36] however, it has not been investigated whether glucose-releasing properties such as the presence of GLUT-2 on the cellular membrane are intact as normal hepatocytes in low-grade HCC cells. Although F-18-FDG-6-phosphate can be dephosphorylated to F-18-FDG in low-grade HCCs by increased G6Pase activity per se, F-18-FDG will be retained in the cytoplasm as in high-grade HCCs unless the glucose-releasing properties are maintained. However, the glucose-releasing mechanisms might be altered even in low-grade HCCs when transmembrane GLUT-2 is replaced by GLUT-1. Otherwise, low uptake of F-18-FDG could be related to low expression of GLUTs, HK IIs, or both, independent of G6Pase activity.

Nevertheless, previous compartmental analysis using a hepatoma cell line or a woodchuck animal model of hepatitis virus–induced HCCs demonstrated that HK activity is increased in a high-grade tumor model, whereas G6Pase activity is decreased,[28,37,38] which support the fact that F-18-FDG uptake is correlated with the histopathologic differentiation of human HCCs and their glycolytic and gluconeogenesis enzyme activities.

Implications of F-18-fluorodeoxyglucose uptake patterns in the prediction of prognosis in hepatocellular carcinomas

Although the sensitivity of F-18-FDG PET scan in HCCs is low, it has an important role in the prediction of prognosis. Insofar as F-18-FDG uptake in HCCs reflects histopathologic differentiation of the tumors, the degree of F-18-FDG uptake can be a prognostic marker. The standardized uptake value (SUV) ratio, expressed as the tumor/nontumor ratio of the SUV, has been reported to be well correlated with tumor volume doubling time and the cumulative survival rate of primary HCCs.[39] A recent article by Seo and colleagues[40] demonstrated that serum alpha-fetoprotein level (risk ratio 8.78; $P = .006$) and tumor/nontumor ratio (risk ratio 1.6; $P = .02$) were independent predictors of survival after resection in multivariate analysis using a Cox proportional hazards model. In addition, F-18-FDG was correlated with the postoperative disease-free survival rate and recurrence. Also, F-18-FDG PET is a useful predictor of survival and tumor recurrence after liver transplant. In Yang and colleagues'[41] study, the 2-year recurrence-free survival rate was significantly higher, and the tumor recurrence rate was lower, in patients who had low FDG uptake after liver transplant.

The underlying pathophysiologic mechanisms of poor prognosis and more aggressive behaviors in HCCs with high FDG uptake could be multifactorial; among them, HK II appears to play a pivotal role. Like many other malignant tumors, HK II is markedly overexpressed in rapidly growing hepatoma cells, and 50% to 80% of total HK IIs are bound to the outer membrane of mitochondria, so it is easier to access mitochondrially generated ATP.[22,42,43] Unlike HK I, each NH2- and COOH-terminal half of HK II has glucose catalytic activity.[44] The overexpressed HK IIs bound to the outer membrane of mitochondria bind both ATP generated from the mitochondria and incoming

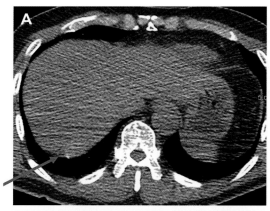
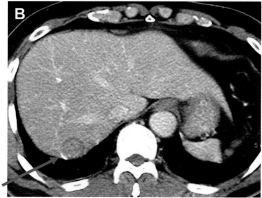
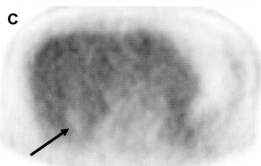

Fig. 3. F-18-FDG PET in a patient who has benign post–inflammatory granuloma. (*A*) Precontrast CT shows a high-density mass in the right lobe of the liver (*arrow*), but (*B*) it is seen as a low-density well-encapsulated mass on postcontrast CT (*arrow*). (*C*) F-18-FDG PET shows photon defect within this mass lesion (*arrow*).

cytosolic glucose; then HK not only produces G6P for energy but also suppresses cancer cell death by interacting with the mitochondrial outer membrane pore (porin), known as the voltage-dependent anion channel (VDAC), which also interacts with adenine nucleotide translocator (ANT).[45,46] HK IIs bound to the porin complex

(HK-VDAC-ANT complex) inhibit Bax or Bak binding to mitochondria and result in inhibition of cytochrome c release, thereby inhibiting tumor cell apoptosis. These antiapoptotic effects of HK IIs are known to be mediated by the serine/threonine kinase Akt and its downstream pathways (**Fig. 4**).[47–49] In addition to the antiapoptotic effects of mitochondrially bound HK IIs, the tricarboxylic acid (TCA) cycle is activated and more ATPs and proteins or fatty acids are generated for the rapidly dividing capability of cells.[50]

The pathophysiologic mechanisms underlying overexpression of HK II in malignant cells are still under investigation. A short segment of the proximal region of HK II promoter contains functionally active response elements for many other transcription factors, such as HIF-1 and the tumor suppressor p53, which have point mutations.[51–53] Therefore, interactions with those transcriptional factors involved in tumor progression and proliferation are thought to be responsible for the overexpression of HK II. HK II activity appears to be a major factor regulating tumor cell proliferation and cell viability as compared with GLUT activity.[54,55]

In addition to the antiapoptotic role of HK IIs, the authors have found altered expression of several genes in HCCs with high FDG uptake that were mostly related to tumor cell adhesion, invasion, spreading, or antitumoral immunity, such as vascular cell adhesion molecule 1, vinexin beta (Src homology 3–containing adaptor molecule-1), core 1 uridine diphosphate galactose: n-acetylgalactosamine-alpha-R-beta 1,3-galactosyltransferase, and lectin-like natural killer cell receptor.[56] Based on these pathophysiologic mechanisms, increased F-18-FDG uptake in HCCs could be a surrogate marker of aggressive behavior and poor clinical outcome.

F-18-fluorodeoxyglucose positron emission tomography/positron emission tomography-CT in the diagnosis and staging of hepatocellular carcinomas

With F-18-FDG PET scan alone, detection of low-grade HCCs is limited. Moreover, the distribution of F-18-FDG uptake is inhomogeneous and variable within the tumor mass; therefore, accurate TNM staging is difficult with F-18-FDG PET alone (**Fig. 5**). Additional delayed imaging (dual–time-point imaging) may improve diagnostic accuracy (**Fig. 6**); however, the incremental value of delayed imaging in HCCs has not been fully evaluated yet.

Instead of F-18-FDG PET alone, PET-CT may be used, and non–contrast-enhanced CT images for attenuation correction could increase the

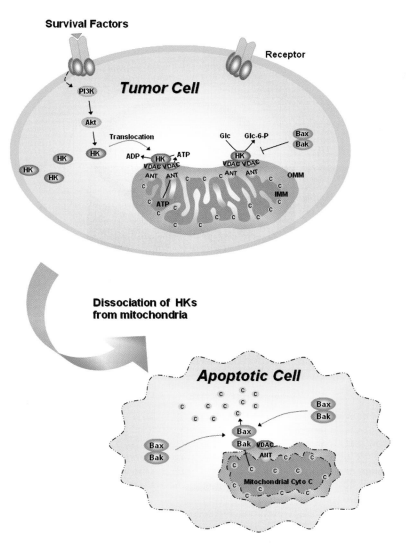

Fig. 4. Antiapoptotic effect of HKs bound to the outer membrane of mitochondria. Activation of phosphatidylinositol 3-kinase (PI3K) by survival factors, such as growth factors, activates the downstream molecular pathway and Akt leads translocation of cytoplasmic HKs to the outer membrane of mitochondria. HKs interact with porin complex (VDAC and ANT) and compete for mitochondrial association of Bax/Bak dimer. Displacement of HKs from the mitochondrial outer membrane facilitates Bax/Bak-mediated cytochrome c release and apoptosis. ADP, adenosine diphophate; Cyto c, cytochrome c; Glc, glucose; Glc-6-p, glucose-6-phosphate; IMM, inner mitochondrial membrane; OMM, outer mitochondrial membrane. (*Modified from* Robey RB, Hay N. Mitochondrial hexokinases, novel mediator of the antiapoptotic effects of growth factors and Akt. Oncogene 2006;25:4683–96; with permission.)

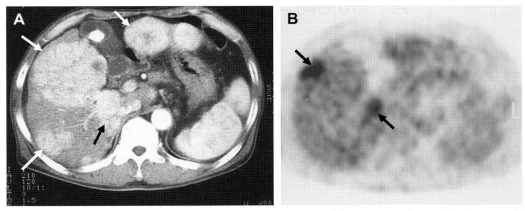

Fig. 5. Inhomogeneous distribution of F-18-FDG within HCC lesions. (*A*) Contrast-enhanced CT shows multiple, variable-sized HCC nodules (*arrows*). (*B*) F-18-FDG uptake is focally increased within the mass lesions (*arrows*).

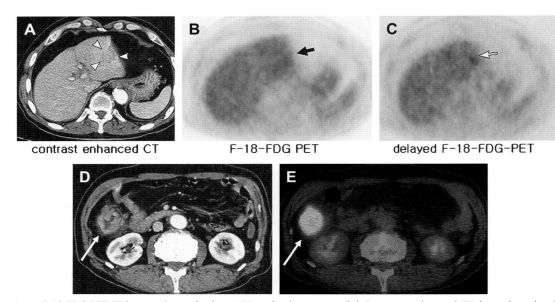

contrast enhanced CT   F-18-FDG PET   delayed F-18-FDG-PET

Fig. 6. F-18-FDG PET-CT in a patient who has HCC and colon cancer. (A) Contrast-enhanced CT shows low-density mass lesion in the lateral segment of the liver (*arrowheads*). (B) F-18-FDG uptake is not significantly increased (*black arrow*), but (C) it can be identified on delayed image (*white arrow*). Dual–time-point imaging may improve the detection rate of low-grade HCCs. In addition, low uptake pattern within the lesion enables the differentiation of HCC from colon cancer metastasis. (D, E) Intense F-18-FDG uptake can be seen within the colon cancer lesion (*arrows*).

detection rate of HCCs, especially in cases showing low F-18-FDG uptake, because approximately 70% of HCCs can be seen on precontrast CT scan as hypointensity (70%), hyperintensity (20%), or isointensity (10%) lesions.[57] However, the image quality of noncontrast low-dose CT for attenuation correction is much poorer than that of precontrast full-dose diagnostic CT; therefore, the detection of HCCs is limited, especially that of small HCCs with conventional PET-CT using noncontrast low-dose CT images. Even multiphase contrast-enhanced full-dose diagnostic CT has a low sensitivity (61%) in HCCs smaller than 2 cm in patients who have cirrhosis, compared with a high sensitivity (93.6%) for lesions larger than 2 cm.[58] Therefore, side-by-side evaluation of PET-CT and conventional diagnostic CT, or obtaining additional full-dose enhanced CT (one of arterial-portal venous or delayed-phase imaging) followed by conventional PET-CT, will increase the detection rate and be useful for the evaluation of tumor extent, especially in portal vein invasion or tumor thrombosis (**Figs. 7** and **8**).

Despite the limitation of F-18-FDG PET in low-grade HCCs, it occasionally makes it easier to differentiate between primary HCCs and liver metastases from F-18-FDG–avid malignancy when dual primary cancers are present in the same patient, as shown in **Fig. 6**.

In metastasis workup, extrahepatic metastasis to the lung (55%), abdominal lymph nodes (LNs) (41%), and bone (28%), and peritoneal seeding are common in patients who have advanced-stage HCC; therefore, staging the workup is necessary to detect metastatic sites correctly.[59] In contrast to its low sensitivity in the detection of intrahepatic HCC lesions, F-18-FDG PET seems to be more accurate in assessing extrahepatic metastasis. In a study that evaluated 19 patients who had HCCs, FDG PET detected metastatic lesions in 5 of 14 patients that were undetected or inconclusive on other studies.[7] In another study, of 20 patients who had HCCs, the sensitivity of F-18-FDG PET for extrahepatic metastasis was 83% and it was also helpful in detecting additional metastases that were not detected on conventional diagnostic workup in 3 patients.[60] In the authors' recent study, the initial TNM stage, based on the conventional staging workup, was changed in 4 of 87 patients after FDG PET.[61] Moreover, Wudel and colleagues[9] reported a higher significant impact in the diagnosis, monitoring, or detection of recurrence in 26 of 91 (28%) patients. Nevertheless, no exact mechanism shows higher sensitivity of F-18-FDG PET in the detection of extrahepatic metastases despite limited sensitivity in the diagnosis of primary intrahepatic HCCs. One possible explanation could be that the degree of F-18-FDG uptake within the primary

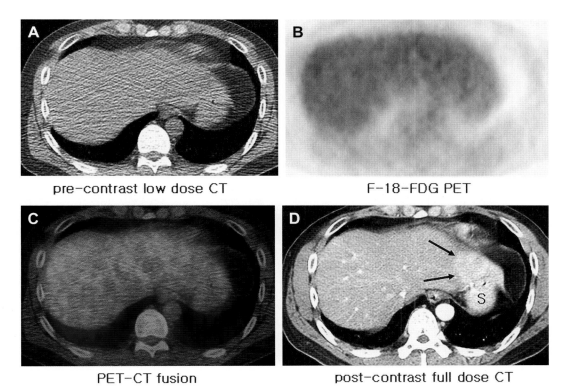

Fig. 7. Low-grade HCC without significant F-18-FDG uptake. Precontrast CT (*A*), F-18-FDG PET (*B*), and PET-CT fusion images (*C*) fail to demonstrate HCC; however, postcontrast CT image (*D*) shows high enhancing mass in the left lobe of the liver (*arrows*) S, stomach.

intrahepatic HCCs is not always parallel to that in the metastatic sites. In some cases, F-18-FDG uptake in the metastatic LNs is higher than that in the primary HCCs (**Fig. 9**), and conversely, low uptake in the metastatic foci, whereas high F-18-FDG uptake in the primary site can be seen (**Fig. 10**). Careful evaluation of CT images on PET-CT will increase the diagnostic accuracy, especially in the detection of pulmonary metastasis, because small lung nodules can easily be overlooked on F-18-FDG PET (**Fig. 11**).

In addition to the usefulness of F-18-FDG PET or PET-CT in the diagnostic workup or prediction of outcome, they are helpful in the evaluation of HCC recurrence after surgical resection, embolization, and radiofrequency ablation therapy. Usually, rim-like hypermetabolic activity persists for 4 to 6 months, surrounding the ablation site after radiofrequency ablation, but a focally increased F-18-FDG uptake could be a tumor recurrence.[62] F-18-FDG PET could also be useful in the detection of tumor recurrence in patients who have unexplained rising alpha-fetoprotein levels after treatment of HCC. The sensitivity, specificity, and accuracy of FDG PET in detecting HCC recurrence were 73.3%, 100%, and 74.2%, respectively in

those circumstances. Therefore, F-18-FDG PET could be a valuable imaging tool in patients who have rising tumor markers and normal conventional examinations.[63]

Fatty acid metabolism and carbon-11-acetate positron emission tomography/positron emission tomography-CT in hepatocellular carcinomas

Fatty acid metabolism is as important as glucose metabolism for cancer cell survival and growth. Fatty acid synthase expression is known to be associated with the prognosis of patients who have cancer. Fatty acids can be derived from acetyl-coenzyme A (CoA). It is converted to malonyl-CoA by acetyl-CoA carboxylase, then to palmitate by fatty acid synthase.[64] Because acetate is believed to be an acetyl donor for the synthesis of acetyl-CoA, C-11-acetate has been evaluated for tumor imaging PET tracer, and it appears to be useful in the evaluation of HCCs not seen on F-18-FDG PET (**Fig. 12**).[10,65]

In terms of C-11-acetate uptake mechanisms, acetyl-CoA can be used either for ATP production by way of the TCA cycle in the mitochondria, or for fatty acid synthesis in the cytoplasm (**Fig. 13**).

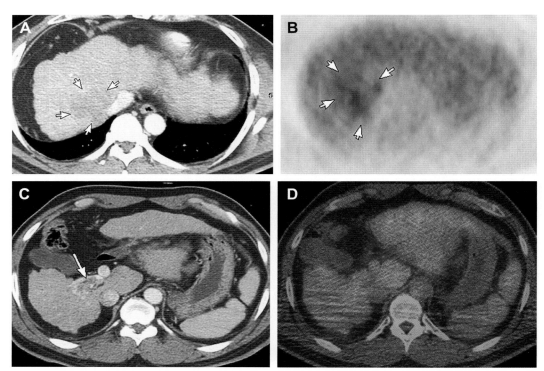

Fig. 8. HCC with portal vein tumor thrombosis. (*A*) Contrast-enhanced CT shows a low-density mass lesion in the right lobe of the liver (*arrows*) and (*B*) F-18-FDG uptake is inhomogeneously increased within the lesion (*arrows*). (*C*) Tumor thrombus is seen in the portal vein (*arrow*) but (*D*) it is difficult to detect on F-18-FDG PET-CT fusion image.

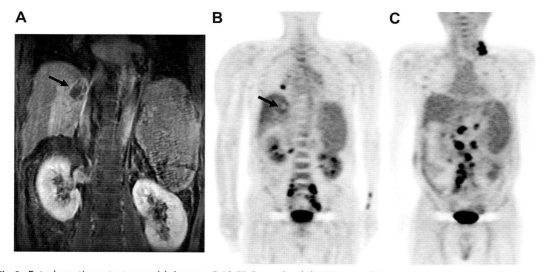

Fig. 9. Extrahepatic metastases with intense F-18-FDG uptake. (*A*) MR coronal image shows a peripherally enhancing HCC in the liver (*arrow*). (*B*) F-18-FDG PET shows mildly increased uptake along the margin of the tumor (*arrow*), but (*B, C*) intense uptake within the metastatic LNs in the retroperitoneum, pelvic LN chain, and left supraclavicular LNs.

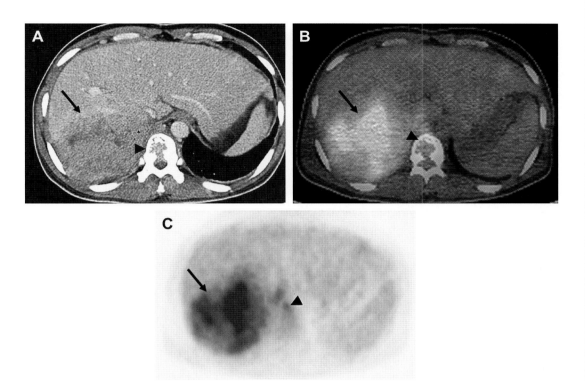

Fig. 10. Intense F-18-FDG uptake within intrahepatic HCC with decreased uptake within metastatic bone lesion. A large HCC mass in the right lobe of the liver (*A, arrow*) shows intense F-18-FDG uptake (*B, arrows*) but uptake is decreased within the osteolytic metastatic bone lesion (*C, arrowheads*).

Recent studies have demonstrated that an animal model of HCC (woodchuck model) showed increased enzyme activity of acetyl-CoA synthetase, which synthesizes acetyl-CoA using acetate, ATP, and CoA, and lipogenic enzymes, including acetyl-CoA carboxylase and fatty acid synthase. It has been demonstrated that radiolabeled acetate incorporated into the triglyceride pool in HepG2 tumor cells.[66–68] Therefore, the preferred uptake mechanisms of C-11-acetate in low-grade HCCs need to be elucidated further, whether it is used for ATP production because of low expression of GLUTs and HKs (low glucose environment) or for fatty acid synthesis.

In a previous study, the sensitivity of C-11-acetate PET in detecting primary HCCs was reported to be much higher than that of F-18-FDG PET, at 87.3% and 47.3%, respectively. C-11-acetate uptake patterns are different from those of F-18-FDG in HCCs. C-11-acetate uptake was increased in low F-18-FDG–uptake HCCs (low-grade HCCs), whereas C-11-acetate uptake was low in HCCs with high F-18-FDG uptake (high-grade HCCs). Unlike HCCs, cholangiocarcinoma or non–HCC-origin metastatic lesions did not show abnormal C-11-acetate uptake.[10] Based on these findings, dual-tracer imaging using C-11-acetate and

F-18-FDG is more effective than single tracer PET/PET-CT imaging in the detection of primary hepatic lesions and metastases. The negative predictive value of dual-tracer imaging was 90% in identifying candidates for curative surgery.[10,69]

As an alternative to C-11-acetate imaging, F-18-fluorocholine (FCH), which is a marker of phosphatidylcholine, an element of phospholipids in the cell membrane, is reported to be an attracting tracer in detecting HCCs. Talbot and colleagues[70] have demonstrated all patients who had primary or recurrent HCCs were detected with F-18-FCH PET, whereas 5 of 9 patients were positive with F-18-FDG PET. Although F-18-FCH PET has a trend toward higher F-18-FCH uptake in low-grade HCCs, the uptake mechanism appears to be different from C-11-acetate, the former incorporated to phospholipids in the cell membrane and the latter incorporated into the triglyceride pool or into the TCA cycle to produce ATP.

Cholangiocarcinoma

Cholangiocarcinoma is an uncommon tumor that originates in intrahepatic or extrahepatic bile ducts. Cholangiocarcinoma is the second most common malignancy in the liver, and comprises

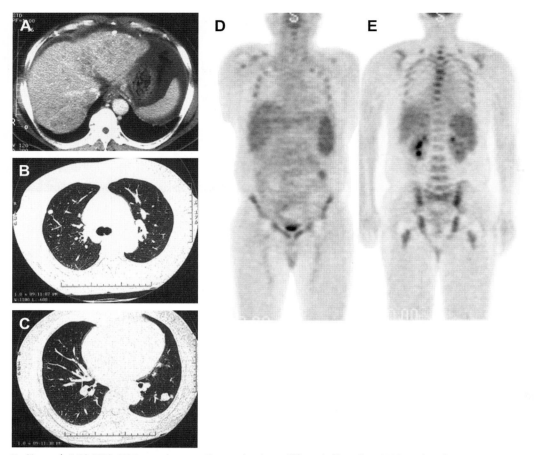

Fig. 11. Normal F-18-FDG PET scan in a patient who has diffuse infiltrating HCC and pulmonary metastases. Contrast-enhanced CT shows diffuse low-density infiltrating HCC lesions (*A*) and multiple metastatic lung nodules (*B*, *C*), but F-18-FDG uptake is not increased (*D*, *E*).

10% to 15% of hepatobiliary malignancies. It can be classified into intrahepatic, hilar, and distal extrahepatic bile duct tumors, according to anatomic location. About 60% to 70% of cholangiocarcinomas arise at the bifurcation of the hepatic ducts (hilar) and 20% to 30% in the distal common bile duct (extrahepatic). Five percent to 10% of cholangiocarcinomas are the peripheral type (intrahepatic), which develops within intrahepatic ducts of the liver parenchyma.[71,72]

F-18-fluorodeoxyglucose uptake patterns with pathologic correlation

The common pathologic finding of cholangiocarcinoma is a well-to-moderately differentiated tubular adenocarcinoma. Mucin is often found in glandular

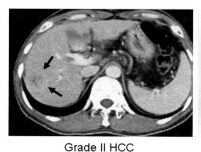

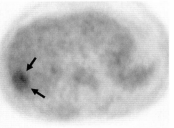

Grade II HCC   F-18-FDG   C-11-acetate

Fig. 12. Comparison of F-18-FDG PET and C-11-acetate PET in a patient who has low-grade HCC (*arrows*).

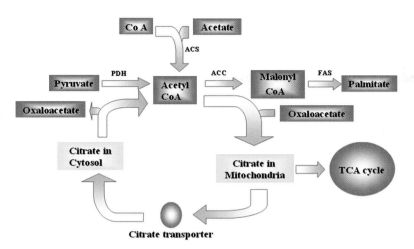

Fig. 13. Acetyl-CoA metabolic pathway. ACC, acetyl-CoA carboxylase; ACs, acetyl-CoA synthetase; FAS, fatty acid synthase; PDH, pyruvate dehydrogenase; TCA, tricarboxylic acid.

lumens that are lined by small cuboidal cells. Most intraductal-growing cholangiocarcinomas are papillary adenocarcinomas.[73]

The Liver Cancer Study Group of Japan has proposed a new classification for intrahepatic cholangiocarcinoma based on growth characteristics: mass-forming, periductal-infiltrating, and intraductal-growing types.[74] Extrahepatic cholangiocarcinoma has been classified into sclerosing, nodular, and papillary phenotypes. Therefore, the

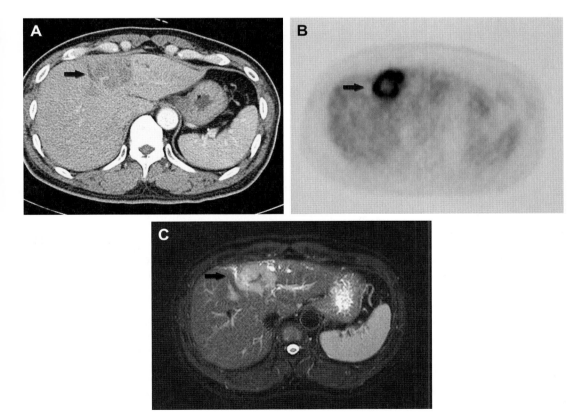

Fig. 14. Intrahepatic mass-forming cholangiocarcinoma. (*A*) Arterial phase CT demonstrates a large low-density mass in the medial segment (*arrow*). (*B*) F-18-FDG PET shows hypermetabolic mass with central hypometabolic core (*arrow*). (*C*) T2-weighted MR imaging shows hyperintense viable tumor with central hypointense fibrotic area (*arrow*).

nodular type matches the mass-forming type, the sclerotic type matches the periductal-infiltrating type, and the papillary type matches the intraductal-type, based on the new classification.[75]

The sensitivity of FDG PET for detecting cholangiocarcinoma varies with the anatomic location and the morphologic type of tumor. The differences in FDG uptakes can be related to the tumor size, the arrangement of fibrous stroma, and the mucin pool in the tumors.

Mass-forming cholangiocarcinoma Most intrahepatic cholangiocarcinomas are of the mass-forming type[76] and extrahepatic or hilar mass-forming cholangiocarcinoma is rare. This type of tumor usually attains a large size before it becomes clinically apparent, because it does not obstruct the central biliary system.

Mass-forming cholangiocarcinoma shows intense F-18-FDG uptake because of increased expression of membranous GLUT-1;[31] however, this type of tumor often produces abundant central desmoplastic reaction and various degrees of fibrosis or necrosis. Therefore, it can be seen as a mass with peripheral hypermetabolism and

central photon defect on F-18-FDG PET (**Fig. 14**), similar to the findings of the peripheral rim-like contrast-enhancement pattern on multiphase contrast-enhanced CT or MR imaging.[77,78]

The F-18-FDG PET sensitivity for intrahepatic mass-forming cholangiocarcinoma depends on the size and the degree of internal fibrosis and necrosis but ranges from 85% to 95%, which is significantly higher than that of CT. The sensitivity of F-18-FDG PET for the mass-forming type is also higher than that for the hilar or extrahepatic periductal-infiltrating types.[79–83]

Periductal-infiltrating cholangiocarcinoma Periductal-infiltrating cholangiocarcinoma is the most common type of hilar and extrahepatic cholangiocarcinoma. Periductal-infiltrating cholangiocarcinoma grows longitudinally along the bile duct, resulting in a diffuse, annular thickening of the extrahepatic bile duct with complete or near-total obstruction of the lumen. Frequently, it involves both intrahepatic and extrahepatic bile ducts.[72,75] This type of tumor becomes symptomatic early because it induces obstructive jaundice.[71] Diffuse wall thickening of the bile ducts, rather than a sizable

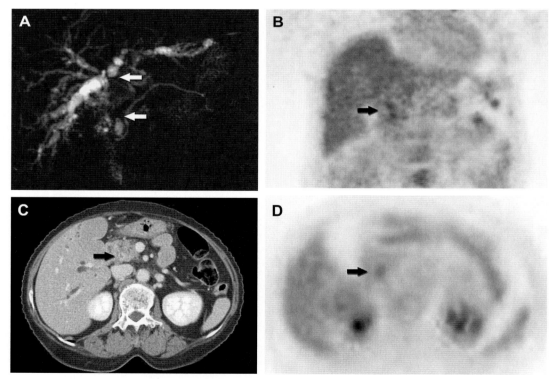

Fig.15. Hilar periductal-infiltrating cholangiocarcinoma. (*A*) MR cholangiopancreatography demonstrates obliteration of the hilar bile ducts (*arrows*). (*B*) F-18-FDG PET coronal image shows nodular lesions along the bile duct with mild hypermetabolism (*arrow*). (*C*) Contrast-enhanced CT shows concentric narrowing and wall thickening with contrast enhancement along the bile duct (*arrow*). (*D*) F-18-FDG PET axial image shows mild FDG uptake in the corresponding lesion (*arrow*).

focal mass, is a major finding.[84] On PET scan, it can be seen as focal, nodular, increased F-18-FDG uptakes, or it may have a linear branching appearance along the biliary tracts (**Fig. 15**).[85]

Because periductal-infiltrating cholangiocarcinoma has only loosely connected cell nests embedded in conspicuous fibrous stroma on histology, sufficient levels of F-18-FDG uptake may not be seen on PET scan because of a lower population of tumor cells but a higher amount of fibrous tissue (**Fig. 16**).[86] Therefore, the sensitivity of F-18-FDG PET for hilar or extrahepatic periductal-infiltrating types ranges from 18% to 69%, and is reported to be lower than that of CT.[79–83]

Acute inflammatory reaction in primary sclerosing cholangitis, which predisposes to cholangiocarcinoma, and in the stent insertion site, may also produce increased F-18-FDG uptake. It makes the differentiation from cholangiocarcinoma difficult. However, nodular increased F-18-FDG uptake on additional delayed (dual–time-point) imaging was reported to be helpful in the differentiation from benign stricture.[87] Similar to dual–time-point imaging, dynamic imaging with net metabolic clearance of F-18-FDG using parametric analysis has been demonstrated to be effective in the differentiation of cholangiocarcinoma in patients who have primary sclerosing cholangitis.[88]

Intraductal-growing cholangiocarcinoma Intrahepatic intraductal-growing cholangiocarcinoma is a low-grade tumor with a better prognosis than other types of cholangiocarcinomas. It is characterized by the presence of intraluminal papillary tumors of the intrahepatic bile ducts with partial obstruction and dilation of the bile ducts. This type of tumor occasionally produces abundant mucin, resulting in a well-marginated cystic mass.[89] Because of its small size and high mucin content, F-18-FDG uptake in this tumor is usually low. Although limited studies focused on F-18-FDG PET sensitivity for intraductal-growing cholangiocarcinoma, a previous study indicated that the SUV of the intraductal-growing type was between the mass-forming type and the periductal-infiltrating type.[90]

Staging with F-18-fluorodeoxyglucose positron emission tomography/positron emission tomography-CT

Because surgical resection of cholangiocarcinoma is a potentially curable treatment modality, imaging studies are used to assess resectability and

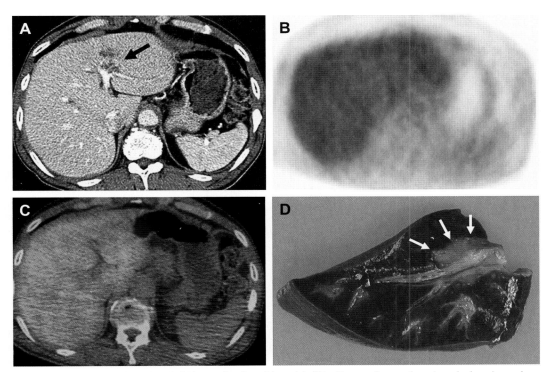

Fig. 16. False-negative F-18-FDG PET-CT in a mixed periductal-infiltrating and mass-forming cholangiocarcinoma. (*A*) Contrast-enhanced CT demonstrates irregular low-density lesion along the left hepatic bile ducts (*arrow*). (*B, C*) F-18-FDG PET axial and fusion images do not show abnormal increased F-18-FDG uptake within this region. (*D*) Gross pathologic specimen shows infiltrating and mass-forming lesion along the bile duct (*arrows*).

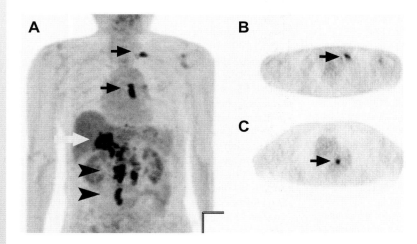

A

B

C

Fig. 17. A mass-forming cholangiocarcinoma with distant metastasis. (*A*) F-18-FDG PET projection image shows intense FDG uptake in the hepatic hilum (*white arrow*) and multiple abdominal LNs (*arrowheads*). F-18-FDG axial image demonstrates metastasis in the left supraclavicular LN (*A, upper arrow; B, arrow*) and mediastinum (*A, lower arrow; C, arrow*).

distant metastasis. In general, metastasis to the celiac, periportal, and superior mesenteric nodes suggests advanced disease and should be considered a contraindication to surgery.[91]

Intrahepatic mass-forming cholangiocarcinoma arises from the mucosa of the bile ducts, grows into the lumen, and penetrates the bile duct wall. Tumor cells have a potential to invade small portal vessels and cause portal vein thrombosis.[92] Extrahepatic spread is common and LN metastasis occurs frequently (**Fig. 17**). Seo and colleagues[93] demonstrated that F-18-FDG PET is superior to CT or MR imaging in the detection of LN metastasis; accuracies were 86%, 68%, and 58%, respectively, in mass-forming intrahepatic cholangiocarcinoma. Although hilar or extrahepatic periductal-infiltrating cholangiocarcinoma does not produce a sizable focal lesion, metastasis to regional and peripancreatic nodes is frequent. Lymphatic metastasis most commonly involves the portocaval, superior pancreaticoduodenal, and posterior pancreaticoduodenal LNs. Retroperitoneal lymphadenopathy, peritoneal spread, and proximal intestinal obstruction occur in advanced stages of hilar cholangiocarcinoma. Kato and colleagues[80] reported that FDG-PET accurately evaluated the LN metastasis in 86% of patients who had extrahepatic cholangiocarcinoma. Detection of unsuspected distant metastases that have been missed by standard imaging is important because it leads to a change in management. F-18-FDG-PET or PET-CT is particularly useful in patients who have intrahepatic cholangiocarcinoma[81,85,94] because of the high incidence of distant metastasis at the time of diagnosis and intense FDG uptake in the intrahepatic cholangiocarcinoma. In previous studies, 17% to 24% of patients underwent treatment change after FDG

PET, mainly because of the detection of distant metastasis.[82,94]

Intraductal-growing cholangiocarcinoma grows and spreads superficially along the bile duct mucosa and does not invade deeply into the fibromuscular layer, and infiltration of the bile duct wall occurs during the late stage; metastasis is rarely observed. Therefore, the role of F-18-FDG PET in evaluating intraductal-growing cholangiocarcinoma appears to be limited.

Detection of recurrence and prognosis prediction with F-18-fluorodeoxyglucose positron emission tomography

In addition to its usefulness in diagnostic workup, F-18-FDG PET is helpful in the evaluation of cholangiocarcinoma recurrence. A previous study demonstrated that the sensitivity and specificity of PET in detecting cholangiocarcinoma recurrence were 94% and 100%, whereas those of CT were 82% and 43%, respectively.[79] As in HCCS, the disease-free survival rates after surgical resection in the high-SUV group were reported to be significantly lower than in the low-SUV group, and a high SUV appears to be an independent predictor of postoperative recurrence.[93]

SUMMARY

F-18-FDG PET/PET-CT is useful in staging, prediction of prognosis, evaluation of recurrence, and treatment response in HCCs and cholangiocarcinomas. Increased F-18-FDG uptake within tumors could be a surrogate marker of aggressive behavior and poor clinical outcome, despite high false-negative rates in detecting primary intrahepatic low-grade HCCs and periductal-infiltrating cholangiocarcinomas. Dual-tracer PET or PET-CT using C-11-acetate and F-18-FDG will increase diagnostic performance in HCC.

REFERENCES

1. Wong R, Corley DA. Racial and ethnic variations in hepatocellular carcinoma incidence within the United States. Am J Med 2008;121:525–31.

2. El-Serag HB, Mason AC. Rising incidence of hepatocellular carcinoma in the United States. N Engl J Med 1999;340:745–50.

3. Tabor E. Hepatocellular carcinoma: global epidemiology. Dig Liver Dis 2001;33:115–7.

4. Schroder O, Trojan J, Zeuzem S, et al. Limited value of fluorine-18-fluorodeoxyglucose PET for the differential diagnosis of focal liver lesions in patients with chronic hepatitis C virus infection. Nuklearmedizin 1998;37:279–85.

5. Delbeke D, Martin WH, Sandler MP, et al. Evaluation of benign vs malignant hepatic lesions with positron emission tomography. Arch Surg 1998;133:510–5.

6. Trojan J, Schroeder O, Raedle J, et al. Fluorine-18 FDG positron emission tomography for imaging of hepatocellular carcinoma. Am J Gastroenterol 1999;94:3314–9.

7. Khan M, Combs C, Brunt E, et al. Positron emission tomography scanning in the evaluation of hepatocellular carcinoma. J Hepatol 2000;32:792–7.

8. Jeng LB, Changlai SP, Shen YY, et al. Limited value of 18F-2-deoxyglucose positron emission tomography to detect hepatocellular carcinoma in hepatitis B virus carriers. Hepatogastroenterology 2003;50:2154–6.

9. Wudel LJ Jr, Delbeke D, Morris D, et al. The role of [18F]fluorodeoxyglucose positron emission tomography imaging in the evaluation of hepatocellular carcinoma. Am Surg 2003;69:117–24.

10. Ho C, Yu S, Yeung D. 11C-acetate PET imaging in hepatocellular carcinoma and other liver masses. J Nucl Med 2003;44:213–21.

11. Raddatz D, Ramadori G. Carbohydrate metabolism and the liver: actual aspects from physiology and disease. Z Gastroenterol 2007;45:51–62.

12. Stumpel F, Brucelin R, Jungermann K, et al. Normal kinetics of intestinal glucose absorption in the absence of GLUT2: evidence for a transport pathway requiring glucose phosphorylation and transfer into the endoplasmic reticulum. Proc Natl Acad Sci U S A 2001;25:11330–5.

13. Ogawa A, Kurita K, Ikezawa Y, et al. Functional localization of glucose transporter 2 in rat liver. J Histochem Cytochem 1996;44:1231–6.

14. Gorovits N, Cui L, Busik JV, et al. Regulation of hepatic GLUT8 expression in normal and diabetic models. Endocrinology 2003;144:1703–11.

15. Postic C, Shiota M, Magnus M. Cell-specific roles of glucokinase in glucose homeostasis. Recent Prog Horm Res 2001;56:195–217.

16. Wilson JE. Isozymes of mammalian hexokinase; structure, subcellular localization and metabolic function. J Exp Biol 2003;206:2049–57.

17. Vaulont S, Munnich A, Decaux JF, et al. Transcriptional and post-transcriptional regulation of L-type pyruvate kinase gene expression in rat liver. J Biol Chem 1986;261:7621–5.

18. Giffhorn-Katz S, Katz NR. Carbohydrate-dependent induction of fatty acid synthase in primary cultures of rat hepatocytes. Eur J Biochem 1986;159:513–8.

19. Argaud D, Kirby TL, Newgard CB, et al. Stimulation of glucose-6-phosphatase gene expression by glucose and fructose-2,6-bisphosphate. J Biol Chem 1997;272:12854–61.

20. Asano T, Katagri H, Tsukuda K, et al. Upregulation of GLUT2 mRNA by glucose, mannose, and fructose in isolated rat hepatocytes. Diabetes 1992;41:22–5.

21. Reneurel F, MunozAlonso MJ, Girad J, et al. An unusual high-Lm hexokinase is expressed in the mhAT3F hepatoma cell line. J Biol Chem 1998;273:26187–93.

22. Rempel A, Mathupala SP, Griffin CA, et al. Glucose catabolism in cancer cells: amplification of the gene encoding type II hexokinase. Cancer Res 1996;56:2468–71.

23. Warburg O. On respiratory impairment in cancer cells. Science 1956;124:269–270.

24. Pedersen PL. Warburg, me and hexokinase 2: multiple discoveries of key molecular events underlying one of cancer's most common phenotypes, the "Warburg effect", i.e., elevated glycolysis in the presence of oxygen. J Bioenerg Biomembr 2007;39:211–22.

25. Dang CV, Semenza GL. Oncogenic alterations of metabolism. Trends Biochem Sci 1999;24:68–72.

26. Minchenko A, Leshchinsky I, Opentanova I, et al. Hypoxia-inducible factor-1-mediated expression of the 6-phosphofructo-2-kinase/fructose-2,6-biphosphatase-3 (PFKFB3) gene. J Biol Chem 2002;277:6183–7.

27. Christofk HR, Vander Heiden MG, Harris MH, et al. The M2 splice isoform of pyruvate kinase is important for cancer metabolism and tumour growth. Nature 2008;452:230–3.

28. Whitesell RR, Ardehali H, Beechem JM, et al. Compartmentalization of transport and phosphorylation of glucose in a hepatoma cell line. Biochem J 2005;386:245–53.

29. Roh MS, Jeong JS, Kim YH, et al. Diagnostic utility of GLUT 1 in the differential diagnosis of liver carcinomas. Hepatogastroenterology 2004;51:1315–8.

30. Zimmerman RL, Fogt F, Burke M, et al. Assessment of Glut-1 expression in cholangiocarcinoma, benign

biliary lesion and hepatocellular carcinoma. Oncol Rep 2002;9:689–92.

31. Lee JD, Yang WI, Park YN, et al. Different glucose uptake and glycolytic mechanisms between hepatocellular carcinoma and intrahepatic mass forming cholangiocarcinoma with increased ^{18}F-fluorodeoxyglucose uptake. J Nucl Med 2005;46:1753–9.

32. Wachsberger PR, Gressen EL, Bhala A, et al. Variability in glucose transporter-1 level and hexokinase activity in human melanoma. Melanoma Res 2002;12:35–43.

33. Aloj L, Caraco C, Jagoda E, et al. GLUT-1 and hexokinase expression: relationship with 2-Fluoro-2-deoxy-D-glucose uptake in A431 and T47D cells in culture. Cancer Res 1999;59:4709–14.

34. Thorens B, Cheng ZQ, Brown D, et al. Liver glucose transporter: a basolateral protein in hepatocytes and intestine and kidney cells. Am J Physiol 1990;259. C279–85.

35. Guillam MT, Brucelin R, Thorens B. Normal hepatic glucose production in the absence of GLUT2 reveals an alternative pathway for glucose release from hepatocytes. Proc Natl Acad Sci U S A 1998;95:12317–21.

36. Torizuka T, Tamaki N, Inokuma T, et al. In vivo assessment of glucose metabolism in hepatocellular carcinoma with FDG-PET. J Nucl Med 1995;36:1811–7.

37. Kuang Y, Schomisch SJ, Chandramouli V, et al. Hexokinase and glucose-6-phosphatase activity in woodchuck model of hepatitis virus-induced hepatocellular carcinoma. Comp Biochem Physiol C Toxicol Pharmacol 2006;143:225–31.

38. Salem N, MacLennan GT, Kuang Y, et al. Quantitative evaluation of 2-Deoxy-2-[F-18]fluoro-D-glucose positron emission tomography imaging on the woodchuck model of hepatocellular carcinoma with histological correlation. Mol Imaging Biol 2007;9:135–43.

39. Shiomi S, Nishiguchi S, Ishizu H, et al. Usefulness of positron emission tomography with fluorine-18-fluorodeoxyglucose for predicting outcome in patients with hepatocellular carcinoma. Am J Gastroenterol 2001;96:1877–80.

40. Seo S, Hatano E, Higashi T, et al. Florine-18 fluorodeoxyglucose positron emission tomography predicts tumor differentiation, P-glycoprotein expression, and outcome after resection in hepatocellular carcinoma. Clin Cancer Res 2007;13:427–33.

41. Yang SH, Suh KS, Lee HW, et al. The role of F-18-FDG-PET imaging for the selection of liver transplantation candidates among hepatocellular carcinoma patients. Liver Transpl 2006;12:1655–60.

42. Bustamante E, Pedersen PL. High aerobic glycolysis of rat hepatoma cells in culture: role of mitochondrial hexokinase. Proc Natl Acad Sci U S A 1997;74:3735–9.

43. Arora KK, Pedersen PL. Functional significance of mitochondrial bound hexokinase in tumor cell metabolism. J Biol Chem 1988;263:17422–8.

44. Ardehali H, Yano Y, Printz RL, et al. Functional organization of mammalian hexokinase II. J Biol Chem 1996;271:1849–52.

45. Vyssokikh M, Brdiczka D. VDAC and peripheral channeling complexes in health and disease. Mol Cell Biochem 2004;256/257:117–26.

46. Shinohara Y, Ishida T, Hino M, et al. Characterization of porin isoforms expressed in tumor cells. Eur J Biochem 2000;267:6067–73.

47. Robey RB, Hay N. Mitochondrial hexokinases, novel mediator of the antiapoptotic effects of growth factors and Akt. Oncogene 2006;25:4683–96.

48. Majewski N, Nogueira V, Robey B, et al. Akt inhibits apoptosis downstream of BID cleavage via a glucose-dependent mechanism involving mitochondrial hexokinases. Mol Cell Biol 2004;24:730–40.

49. Mathupala SP, Ko YH, Pedersen PL. Hexokinase II: cancer's double-edged sword acting as both facilitator and gatekeeper of malignancy when bound to mitochondria. Oncogene 2006;25:4777–86.

50. Golshani-Heboni SG, Bessman SP. Hexokinase binding to mitochondria: a basis for proliferative energy metabolism. J Bioenerg Biomembr 1997;29:331–8.

51. Mathupala SP, Heese C, Pedersen PL. Glucose catabolism in cancer cells. The type II hexokinase promoter contains functionally active response elements for the tumor suppressor p53. J Biol Chem 1997;36:22776–80.

52. Lee MG, Pedersen PL. Glucose metabolism in cancer. Importance pf transcription factor-DNA interactions within a short segment of the proximal region of the type II hexokinase promoter. J Biol Chem 2003;42:41047–68.

53. Mathupala SP, Hempel A, Pedersen PL. Glucose catabolism in cancer cells. Identification and characterization of a marked activation response of the type II hexokinase gene to hypoxic conditions. J Biol Chem 2001;46:43407–12.

54. Yamada K, Brink I, Bisse E, et al. Factors in influencing [F-18]2-fluoro-2-deoxy-D-glucose (F-18-FDG) uptake in melanoma cells: the role of proliferation rate, viability, glucose transporter expression and hexokinase activity. J Dermatol 2005;32:316–34.

55. Tohma T, Okazuma S, Makino H, et al. Relationship between glucose transporter, hexokinase and FDG-PET in esophageal cancer. Hepatogastroenterology 2005;52:486–90.

56. Lee JD, Yun M, Lee JM, et al. Analysis of gene expression profiles of hepatocellular carcinomas with regard to ^{18}F-fluorodeoxyglucose uptake pattern on positron emission tomography. Eur J Nucl Med Mol Imaging 2004;31:1621–30.

57. Iannaccone R, Placentini F, Murakami T, et al. Hepatocellular carcinoma in patients with nonalcoholic fatty liver disease: helical CT and MR imaging findings with clinical-pathologic comparison. Radiology 2007;243:422–30.

58. Valls C, Cos M, Figueras J, et al. Pretransplantation diagnosis and staging of hepatocellular carcinoma in patients with cirrhosis: value of dual-phase helical CT. Am J Roentgenol 2004;182:1011–7.

59. Katyal S, Oliver JH, Peterson MS, et al. Extrahepatic metastases of hepatocellular carcinoma. Radiology 2000;216:698–703.

60. Sugiyama M, Sakahara H, Torizuka T, et al. ^{18}F-FDG PET in the detection of extrahepatic metastases from hepatocellular carcinoma. J Gastroenterol 2004;39:961–8.

61. Yoon KT, Kim JK, Kim do Y, et al. Role of ^{18}F-fluorodeoxyglucose positron emission tomography in detecting extrahepatic metastasis in pretreatment staging of hepatocellular carcinoma. Oncology 2007;72(Suppl 1):104–10.

62. McGahan JP, Khaltri VP. Imaging findings after liver resection by using radiofrequency parenchymal coagulation devices: initial experiences. Radiology 2008;247:869–902.

63. Chen YK, Hsieh DS, Liao CS, et al. Utility of FDG-PET for investigating unexplained serum AFP elevation in patients with suspected hepatocellular carcinoma recurrence. Anticancer Res 2005;25:4719–25.

64. Kuhajda FP. Fatty acid synthase and cancer: new application of an old pathway. Cancer Res 2006;66:5977–80.

65. Vavere AL, Kridel SJ, Wheeler PB, et al. 1-11C-acetate as a PET radiopharmaceutical for imaging fatty acid synthase expression in prostate cancer. J Nucl Med 2008;49:327–34.

66. Kuang Y, Salem N, Wang F, et al. A colorimetric assay method to measure acetyl-CoA synthetase activity: application to woodchuck model of hepatitis virus-induced hepatocellular carcinoma. J Biochem Biophys Methods 2007;70:649–53.

67. Sugimoto Y, Naniwa Y, Nakamura T, et al. A novel acetyl-CoA carboxylase inhibitor reduces de novo fatty acid synthesis in HepG2 cells and rat primary hepatocytes. Arch Biochem Biophys 2007;468:44–8.

68. Yahagi N, Shimano H, Hasegawa K, et al. Co-ordinate activation of lipogenic enzymes in hepatocellular carcinoma. Eur J Cancer 2006;41:1316–22.

69. Ho CL, Chen S, Yeung DWC, et al. Dual-tracer PET/CT imaging in evaluation of metastatic hepatocellular carcinoma. J Nucl Med 2007;48:902–9.

70. Talbot JN, Gultman F, Fartoux L, et al. PET/CT in patients with hepatocellular carcinoma using ^{18}F]fluorocholine: preliminary comparison with ^{18}F]PET/CT. Eur J Nucl Med Mol Imaging 2006;33:1285–9.

71. Nakeeb A, Pitt HA, Sohn TA, et al. Cholangiocarcinoma. A spectrum of intrahepatic, perihilar, and distal tumors. Ann Surg 1996;224:463–73.

72. Han JK, Choi BI, Kim AY, et al. Cholangiocarcinoma: pictorial essay of CT and cholangiographic findings. Radiographics 2002;22:173–87.

73. Yoon KH, Han HK, Kim CG, et al. Malignant papillary neoplasms of intrahepatic bile ducts: CT and histopathologic features. Am J Roentgenol 2000;175:1135–9.

74. Liver cancer study group of Japan. The general rules for the clinical and pathological study of primary liver cancer. 4th edition. Tokyo: Kanehara; 2000.

75. Lim JH. Cholangiocarcinoma: morphologic classification according to growth pattern and imaging findings. Am J Roentgenol 2003;181:819–27.

76. Soyer P, Bluemke DA, Reichle R, et al. Imaging of intrahepatic cholangiocarcinoma. 1. Peripheral cholangiocarcinoma. Am J Roentgenol 1995;165:1427–31.

77. Kim SJ, Lee JM, Han JK, et al. Peripheral mass-forming cholangiocarcinoma in cirrhotic liver. Am J Roentgenol 2007;189:1428–34.

78. Maetani Y, Itoh K, Watanabe C, et al. MR imaging of intrahepatic cholangiocarcinoma with pathologic correlation. Am J Roentgenol 2001;176:1499–507.

79. Jadvar H, Henderson RW, Conti PS, et al. [F-18]fluorodeoxyglucose positron emission tomography and positron emission tomography: computed tomography in recurrent and metastatic cholangiocarcinoma. J Comput Assist Tomogr 2007;31:223–8.

80. Kato T, Tsukamoto E, Kuge Y, et al. Clinical role of (18)F-FDG PET for initial staging of patients with extrahepatic bile duct cancer. Eur J Nucl Med Mol Imaging 2002;29:1047–54.

81. Anderson CD, Rice MH, Pinson CW, et al. Fluorodeoxyglucose PET imaging in the evaluation of gallbladder carcinoma and cholangiocarcinoma. J Gastrointest Surg 2004;8:90–7.

82. Corvera CU, Blumgart LH, Akhurst T, et al. 18F-fluorodeoxyglucose positron emission tomography influences management decisions in patients with biliary cancer. J Am Coll Surg 2008;206:57–65.

83. Moon CM, Bang S, Chung JB, et al. Usefulness of 18F-fluorodeoxyglucose positron emission tomography in differential diagnosis and staging of cholangiocarcinomas. J Gastroenterol Hepatol 2008;23:759–65.

84. Lim JH, Park CK. Pathology of cholangiocarcinoma. Abdom Imaging 2004;29:540–7.

85. Kim YJ, Yun M, Lee WJ, et al. Usefulness of 18F-FDG PET in intrahepatic cholangiocarcinoma. Eur J Nucl Med Mol Imaging 2003;30:1467–72.

86. de Groen PC, Gores GJ, LaRusso NF, et al. Biliary tract cancers. N Engl J Med 1999;341:1368–78.

87. Reinhardt MJ, Strunk H, Gerhardt T, et al. Detection of Klatskin's tumor in extrahepatic bile duct strictures using delayed ^{18}F-FDG PET/CT: preliminary results for 22 patient study. J Nucl Med 2005;46: 1158–63.

88. Prytz H, Keiding S, Björnsson E, et al. Dynamic FDG-PET is useful for detection of cholangiocarcinoma in patients with PSC listed for liver transplantation. Hepatology 2006;44:1572–80.

89. Guglielmi A, Ruzzenente A, Iacono C. Diagnosis. In: Surgical treatment of hilar and intrahepatic cholangiocarcinoma. Milan, Italy: Springer; 2007. p. 187–92.

90. Nishiyama Y, Yamamoto Y, Kimura N, et al. Comparison of early and delayed FDG PET for evaluation of biliary stricture. Nucl Med Commun 2007;28:914–9.

91. Slattery JM, Sahani DV. What is the current state-of-the-art imaging for detection and staging of cholangiocarcinoma? Oncologist 2006;11:913–22.

92. Sasaki A, Aramaki M, Kawano K, et al. Intrahepatic peripheral cholangiocarcinoma: mode of spread and choice of surgical treatment. Br J Surg 1998; 85:1206–9.

93. Seo S, Hatano E, Higashi T, et al. Fluorine-18-fluorodeoxyglucose positron emission tomography predicts lymph node metastasis, P-glycoprotein expression, and recurrence after resection in mass-forming intrahepatic cholangiocarcinoma. Surgery 2008;143:769–77.

94. Petrowsky H, Wildbrett P, Husarik DB, et al. Impact of integrated positron emission tomography and computed tomography on staging and management of gall bladder cancer and cholangiocarcinoma. J Hepatol 2006;45:43–50.

Liver Metastases

Roland Hustinx, MD, PhD[a],*, Nancy Witvrouw, MD[a],
Tino Tancredi, MD[b]

KEYWORDS

- FDG • PET • PET/CT • Liver metastases
- Gastrointestinal cancers • MR imaging • CT

The liver is the most frequent site of hematogenous metastatic spread, and metastases represent the most frequent liver malignancy in the United States and Europe. Tumors of the gastrointestinal tract, in particular colorectal cancer, are the primary source of metastatic liver involvement but other tumors such as breast and lung cancers and melanomas also present a high likelihood of hepatic dissemination.[1] Close to 50% of the patients with colorectal cancer develop liver metastases, either at initial presentation or during the course of the disease, and the liver is the only site of distant spread in 30% to 50% of these patients. This represents a population that is likely to benefit from local therapy, in particular surgery. Indeed, surgical resection of liver metastases with curative intent can be performed with acceptable morbidity and leads to long-term survival rates of up to 58%. The classical criteria for selecting patients for surgery include the number and size of lesions as well as the necessity to achieve resection with a 1-cm free margin. In addition, the disease has typically to be limited to the liver. Recently, a trend has emerged to expand the inclusion criteria. This can be achieved through combining resection with radiofrequency ablation or neoadjuvant chemotherapy, which aims at reducing the tumor volume to be resected, or through portal vein embolization or two-stage hepatectomy, which aims at increasing the hepatic reserve. As thoroughly discussed in a recent review by Pawlik and colleagues,[2] a new paradigm consists of focusing the surgical decision on what would remain after resection, instead of what is to be removed. Basically, eligibility criteria become all patients in whom all the lesions can be removed, including those outside of the liver, and in whom the hepatic reserve is adequate. Such approach obviously requires multidisciplinary and multimodality collaboration to appropriately select an ever-increasing number of patients. New treatment modalities also involve nuclear medicine physicians, with the development of techniques such as selective internal irradiation of glass or resin microspheres labeled with ^{90}Y.[3,4] Surgical resection of liver metastases from noncolorectal malignancies is also increasingly proposed, although with more limited clinical results and in a smaller number of patients.[5]

CONVENTIONAL IMAGING MODALITIES
Ultrasonography

Transabdominal ultrasonography (US) presents several advantages, including low cost, absence of irradiation, wide availability, and portability. The sensitivity is very low, however, as half of the lesions are missed and the specificity is not very high either.[6] More recently, developments in the technique such as Power Doppler or contrast enhancement with microbubbles have been reported to significantly improve the diagnostic accuracy, which may reach values close to those obtained with CT. For instance, a multicenter study was recently performed in 102 patients with various primaries.[7] Contrast-enhanced US (ceUS) identified 55 lesions classified as metastases, compared with 61 with triple-phase spiral CT and 53 with MR imaging. These results and others[8,9] are encouraging but it should be kept in mind that

[a] Division of Nuclear Medicine, University Hospital of Liège, Campus Universitaire du Sart Tilman B35, 4000 Liège, Belgium
[b] Department of Medical Imaging, University Hospital of Liège, Campus Universitaire du Sart Tilman B35, 4000 Liège, Belgium
* Corresponding author.
E-mail address: rhustinx@chu.ulg.ac.be (R. Hustinx).

PET Clin 3 (2008) 187–195
doi:10.1016/j.cpet.2008.09.004
1556-8598/08/$ – see front matter © 2008 Elsevier Inc. All rights reserved.

ceUS highly depends on the operator's skills and experience. Currently, US is not recommended as a screening or surveillance method for evaluating liver metastases.

CT

CT technology has benefited from major technological improvements over the past decade. Multidetector scanners allow very fast imaging, thus eliminating any respiratory artifacts and allowing precise timing of the various tissue enhancement after intravenous contrast injection, while achieving exquisite spatial resolution in all three planes. The CT appearance of liver metastases varies according to the pathologic type of the primary tumor. Metastases from melanomas, sarcomas, neuroendocrine tumors, and renal cell carcinomas are hypervascular and therefore better visualized during the hepatic arterial phase. Metastases from colorectal cancer are hypovascular and therefore better visualized during the portal venous phase.[10] Although breast cancer metastases may show early arterial enhancement, adding the early phase to the portal phase CT did not improve the sensitivity of the technique.[11] Therefore, triple-phase CT may not be mandatory in most patients being screened for liver metastases.

As may be expected and in spite of a very high spatial resolution, the detection rate of liver metastases by CT shows a negative correlation with the size of the lesions.[12] In lesion-per-lesion analyses, sensitivities ranging from 49% to 89% have been reported.[12–14] The specificity is usually high, although the study that showed the highest sensitivity (89%) also showed a rather poor specificity (67%).[14]

MR Imaging

Similar to CT, MR imaging technology has witnessed important developments, in the hardware, image acquisition protocols, and contrast agents. On non–contrast-enhanced MR imaging, most metastases appear as hypo- to isointense on T1-weighted images and iso- to hyperintense on T2-weighted images.[15] Dynamic imaging after enhancement with gadolinium (Gd)-based agents provides information regarding the vascularity of the lesions and therefore increases the performance of MR imaging for differentiating benign from malignant lesions. Tissue-specific contrast agents have been introduced to increase the tumor-to-liver contrast. Mangafodipir trisodium (MnDPDP, Teslascan) is taken up by the hepatocytes, therefore increasing the signal from the normal liver on T1-weighted images. Superparamagnetic iron oxide (SPIO) is taken up by the reticuloendothelial system (Kupffer cells in the liver) and causes a signal loss on T2-weighted images, therefore darkening the normal liver background on these images. Few systematic studies were performed comparing these tissue-specific contrast agents. In two Korean series from different investigators, the detection rate was similar for both mangafodipir and SPIO MR imaging.[16,17] MnDPDP-MR imaging appears to be more sensitive than both unenhanced MR imaging and spiral CT for detecting individual lesions.[18] Similarly, both Gd-enhanced and SPIO-enhanced MR imaging are more accurate than CT, and SPIO tends to perform better than Gd for detecting subcentimetric lesions.[19] Another series, however, reports similar results for CT and SPIO-enhanced MR imaging.[14] Currently, gadolinium remains the most widely used contrast agent when performing liver MR imaging in the clinical setting, but the precise clinical indication as well as the local experience of the radiology team contribute to guiding the choice of the technique, acquisition sequences, and contrast agent. In particular, MR imaging with liver-specific contrast agents is increasingly recommended in preoperative patients.[20]

PET

Considering that 2-[^{18}F]fluoro-2′-deoxyglucose (FDG) is avidly taken up by most cancer types and given the high prevalence of metastatic spread to the liver, it seems only logical to propose FDG-PET as a diagnostic and staging tool for liver involvement. The feasibility of the technique was suggested by Yonekura and colleagues[21] more than 25 years ago. Further studies, including those performed without attenuation correction, reported in the late 1990s diagnostic performances that compared favorably with the imaging methods routinely used at that time.[22–25] A first meta-analysis comparing US, CT, MR imaging, and PET for detecting liver metastases from cancers of the gastrointestinal tract was published in 2002.[26] The authors analyzed 54 studies, including 9 for US, 25 for CT, 11 for MR imaging, and 9 for PET. The most recent articles were published in 1996 for US and in 2000 for the other techniques. The total number of patients was 509 (US), 1371 (CT), 401 (MR imaging), and 423 (PET). The primaries were colorectal cancers in all cases for PET and MR imaging, and in 74% and 78% for US and CT, respectively. The other primaries were gastric or esophageal cancers. The prevalence of hepatic metastases in the population samples ranged from 33% (US studies) to 58% (PET studies). The mean weighted sensitivity was 66% for US, 70% for

CT, 71% for MR imaging, and 90% for PET. The authors further analyzed the data by stratifying subsets according to specificity. They considered that for any technique to be clinically useful and relevant, its specificity should be superior or equal to 85%. With such a cutoff for specificity, the sensitivity values became 55% for US, 72% for CT, 76% for MR imaging, and 90% for PET. The sensitivity was significantly higher for PET than for US and CT, and marginally higher when compared with MR imaging (*P* = .055). There were statistically significant differences among the sensitivity of all three radiological techniques. Somewhat surprisingly, technical parameters did not influence the sensitivity of the various techniques. For instance, spiral CT did not perform any better than nonspiral CT, and SPIO-enhanced MR imaging was not more sensitive than unenhanced MR imaging. Equally troubling is the observation that in spite of a 15-year range of publication, the detection rate was not higher in the most recent studies, eg, reporting on the most recent technology.

Another meta-analysis was published more recently[27] Sixty-one studies published between January 1990 and December 2003 were included in this review. Only patients with colorectal cancer were considered, and US was not included in the analysis, owing to its well-known low sensitivity for detecting metastases on lesion-per-lesion basis. Overall, 2586 patients were studied with CT (621 with spiral CT), 564 patients with MR imaging (391 with 1.5-T systems), and 1058 with FDG-PET. According to the per-patient analysis, PET was significantly more sensitive (94.6%) than spiral CT (64.7%) and 1.5-T MR imaging (75.8%). The sensitivities for detecting individual lesions (per-lesion analysis) followed a similar pattern, with 63.8% for spiral CT, 64.4% for 1.5-T MR imaging, and 75.9% for FDG-PET. Further analyses showed that Gd and SPIO-enhanced MR imaging performed better than both unenhanced MR imaging and spiral CT with a low amount of contrast media. One limitation of this study is the lack of information regarding the specificity of the various imaging techniques.

Wiering and colleagues[28] further analyzed the performance of FDG-PET and evaluated its clinical impact in the management of colorectal liver metastases. The authors reviewed 32 articles and calculated the lesion-based sensitivity and specificity for detecting liver metastases. Overall, the pooled sensitivity was 88% for PET and 82.7% for CT, and the pooled specificity was 96.1% for PET and 84.1% for CT. When considering only the six studies with the highest methodological score, ie, with the strongest level of evidence, the sensitivity was a bit lower for PET (79.9%) but the specificity remained very high, at 92.3%. CT had a sensitivity of 85.8% and a specificity of 88.3%. These results further illustrate that the diagnostic performances of PET and CT may be considered very similar for detecting individual liver lesions. Worth mentioning is the excellent specificity of PET, as most of the focal lesions that can be mistaken as metastases with CT, such as angiomas or adenomas, do not take up FDG. PET modified the clinical management in 30.8% of the patients in the studies that ranked above the mean regarding the methodological quality and in 25.4% of the patients when the evaluation was limited to the six highest-ranking publications. Most of the management changes came from the higher accuracy of PET for detecting extrahepatic disease. A recent prospective study conducted by the same group in 131 colorectal cancer patients who underwent surgery confirmed that the sensitivity of both PET and CT was a function of the lesions' size. Indeed, only 16% of the 63 metastases smaller than 1 cm were identified with both PET and CT, whereas CT and PET detected 72% and 75%, respectively, of the 123 lesions of 1 to 2 cm and almost all lesions larger than 2 cm were detected with both techniques.[29]

The clinical impact of PET was further emphasized in a series of 100 patients who underwent liver surgery with curative intent for metastatic spread from colorectal cancer.[30] These were preoperatively screened with FDG-PET, so that the operability criteria included the metabolic findings. The actuarial 5-year survival in this group was 58%, which is significantly higher than the 25% survival rate attained when conventional methods are used. In addition, preliminary data suggest that the metabolic activity of the liver metastases may predict the long-term outcome of patients who undergo curative surgery. In a homogeneous series of 90 patients, Riedl and colleagues[31] found that a higher standardized uptake value (SUV) was correlated with a shorter survival, as well as with biological markers such Ki67 and P53 expression.

PET/CT

Despite excellent clinical results with FDG PET, the technique is intrinsically limited by the lack of precise and reliable anatomic information. Foci of increased uptake that are clearly located in the liver parenchyma are readily identified and usually correspond to metastases, but the bowel uptake is highly variable and may be focally increased in regions close to the liver, and therefore be mistaken with peripheral liver lesions. Combined PET/CT scanners allow the precise localization of the abnormal areas of uptake, and thus greatly increase the confidence with which the PET reports are redacted and decreases the proportion of indeterminate or inconclusive findings.[32] Furthermore, modern PET/CT devices are equipped with high-end CT scanners, fully capable of performing full diagnostic CT studies. This raises several questions, such as, how does unenhanced PET/CT (PET/CT) perform compared with standalone PET and ceCT, should contrast-enhanced PET/CT (PET/ceCT) be the preferred modality for evaluating liver metastases, and which role remains for contrast-enhanced CT (ceCT) in the era of PET/CT? These questions are not fully answered yet, but enlightening data were recently published.

PET/CT versus PET, contrast-enhanced CT, and MR imaging

Selzner and colleagues[33] studied 76 patients with liver metastases from colorectal cancer and who were considered for surgery. PET/CT and ceCT were performed within 2 weeks of each other, and results were compared with either surgical findings or clinical follow-up. Both techniques showed similar sensitivities for detecting liver metastases (95% for ceCT, 91% for PET/CT). Ten patients were free of malignant liver involvement. ceCT correctly identified 7 of 10 patients and PET/CT 9 of 10, the lone false-positive result corresponding to an abscess. Interestingly, PET/CT was more specific than ceCT for diagnosing intrahepatic recurrences in patients with prior hepatic resection (100% and 50%, respectively). This observation is clinically relevant, considering the increasing number of patients who undergo iterative liver surgery. The authors further confirmed the added value of PET/CT in detecting extrahepatic lesions, and found an overall positive impact of PET/CT on the clinical management in 21% of the cases. Rappeport and colleagues[14] systematically performed PET/CT, dual-phase ceCT and SPIO-MR imaging in 35 colorectal cancer patients, including 31 who underwent surgery. Both ceCT and MR imaging were significantly more sensitive than PET and PET/CT in a lesion-per-lesion analysis. In a patient-per-patient analysis, the sensitivity was 100% for ceCT, MR imaging, and PET/CT and 92% for PET, when the patients who had a recent chemotherapy were excluded. Indeed, it is well known that the sensitivity of FDG-PET is decreased by chemotherapy,[33] in particular, quite obviously, in patients who respond to the treatment.[34] Overall, the specificity was 99% for PET and PET/CT, 67% for ceCT and 81% for MR imaging.

In yet another effort to clarify the relative performances of all imaging modalities, Kong and colleagues[35] performed PET/CT, ceCT, and MnDPDP-MR imaging in 65 patients with colorectal cancer and known or suspected liver metastases. The gold standard was histopathology in 23 cases and a median clinical follow-up of 13 months in the remaining cases. According to the per-patient analysis, both PET/CT and MR imaging performed equally well, with a sensitivity of 98% and a specificity of 100%. The per-lesion analysis showed a slightly higher sensitivity with MR imaging (99%, 163 lesions detected) than with PET/CT (94%, 155 lesions). Almost all the lesions missed with PET/CT were smaller than 1 cm, which confirms the value of MR imaging for diagnosing small metastases. In 85% of the cases, both methods were concordant regarding the number of liver lesions that were detected. Although these authors compared PET/CT and MR imaging for liver imaging, they compared PET/CT and ceCT for the extrahepatic staging only. Chua et al,[36] however, evaluated PET/CT and ceCT in 131 patients with various malignancies, including 75 with colorectal cancer. All patients had either known or suspected liver involvement. The analysis was performed retrospectively and on a patient-per-patient basis, the gold standard being histology or a 6-month minimum follow-up. PET/CT and ceCT were in agreement in 75.5% of the patients (99 of 131). The sensitivity was 96% and 88%, and the specificity was 75% and 25% for PET/CT and ceCT, respectively. The specificity values must be read with caution, as only less than 10% of the population (12 of 131) was actually free of liver metastases. In addition, 15% of the patients were referred for evaluating indeterminate findings on CT, which may further contribute decreasing the specificity of ceCT. Nonetheless, these results confirm the very high sensitivity of PET/CT for detecting liver metastases, including those arising from noncolorectal tumors. Typical FDG PET/CT studies are shown in **Figs. 1** and **2**.

Diagnostic Algorithms

It clearly appears that a single imaging modality cannot be proposed to answer all the clinical questions that may arise in all patients. The choice among the various techniques, and the sequence with which they are used, should be guided primarily by the clinical indication, taking into account the primary type and the different possible treatments, which also depend on the general status of clinical history of the patient. Nevertheless, according to the results presented in the previous section, it becomes increasingly difficult to defend the role of ceCT in the evaluation of liver metastases. All the available data yield similar conclusions, ie, a sensitivity that is comparable or higher and a specificity that is consistently higher with PET/CT than with ceCT. A positive clinical impact of PET/CT is reported in about 20% to 25% of the cases, primarily by detecting extrahepatic lesions,[33,35] but also by detecting additional liver lesions or even by ruling out liver metastases.[36] On the other hand, Soyka and colleagues[37] recently reported additional information revealed by PET/ceCT as compared with PET/CT in 39 (72%) of 52 patients with recurrent colorectal cancer. This additional information altered the therapeutic management in 23 cases. However, most of these changes came from a proper segmental localization of the liver lesions, which is mandatory before surgery and cannot be reliably provided without intravenous (IV) contrast. As PET/CT, as a whole-body imaging method, is highly accurate

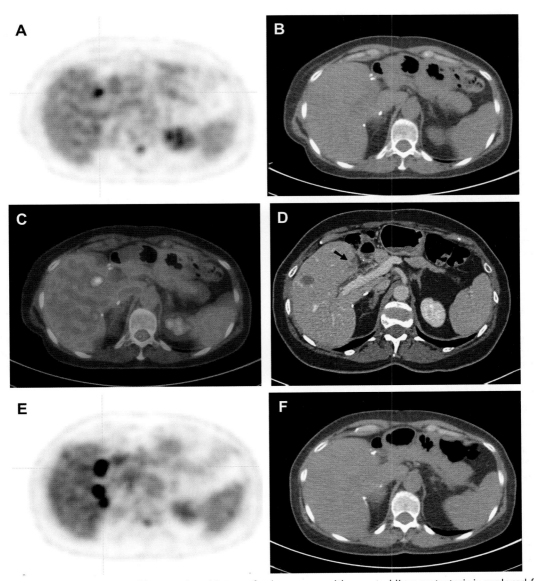

Fig. 1. A 60-year-old woman with a previous history of colon cancer with resected liver metastasis is explored for an increase in CEA levels. The PET/CT shows a small focus of increased activity in the segment IV of the liver (*A*, PET; *B*, low-dose, unenhanced CT; *C*, fused images). The contrast-enhanced CT shows a small lesion, which was already seen on previous CT studies and appears to be stable (*D*, portal phase). The MR imaging is negative. It is thus decided to follow the patients. A repeat PET/CT is performed 4 months later showing a progression of the lesions as well as additional liver metastases (*E–G*). At that time, CeCT and MR imaging confirm the metastatic progression (*H*, portal-phase CT; *I*, Gd-enhanced T1-weighted MR; *J*, T2-weighted MR).

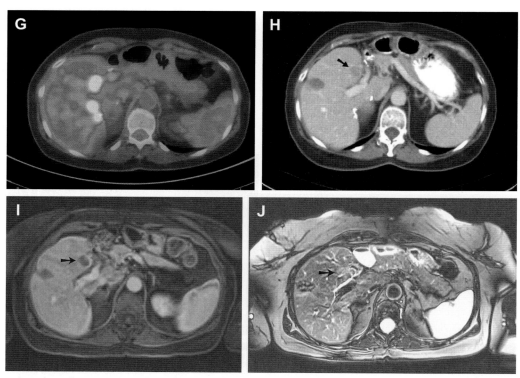

Fig. 1. (continued)

for both the liver and other possible locations of metastatic spread, it seems fairly logical to propose this technique relatively early on in patients who should be selected for a high likelihood of disease, based on clinical criteria. Dedicated liver imaging is not needed in patients diagnosed at PET/CT with disseminated, inoperable disease, whereas both ceCT and MR imaging with tissue-specific contrast agents should complement the preoperative local staging. Cost and availability have often been put forward to prevent PET and PET/CT from being used as a first-line tool. However, cost has significantly decreased and availability, increased, over the past 10 years. Modern scanners are much faster, allowing high throughput while maintaining the radiation burden to the patients within reasonable limits. Of course, this potential algorithm must be appropriately tested and validated, but the matter of the fact is currently that ceCT adds very little, if any, to PET/CT in most patients who are explored for possible liver metastases.

PET/CT and Locoregional Treatment of Liver Metastases

As mentioned earlier, a variety of local ablative therapies are available and may be performed when surgery is contraindicated. These techniques include radiofrequency ablation (RFA), which is the best known, interstitial laser therapy, and microwave ablation. PET/CT has been evaluated in the preinterventional setting, with results very similar to ceCT,[38] but its real value probably lies in the follow-up of patients who underwent such procedure. Several retrospective studies showed, in a limited number of patients, a high accuracy for PET in detecting residual of recurrent lesions after RFA.[39,40] Travaini and colleagues[41] performed in a series of nine patients, both PET/CT and ceCT at 1, 3, 6, and 9 months after RFA. In 7 of 9 patients, PET/CT was positive earlier than ceCT, 3 months on average, for detecting evolutive disease. Kuehl and colleagues[42] showed very similar diagnostic performances for both PET/ceCT and Gd-enhanced MR imaging in 16 patients with metastases from colorectal cancer, with an accuracy of 92% and 91%, respectively. PET/CT was performed as early as 24 hours after ablation. The technique may therefore be proposed as a first-line tool in the follow-up of these patients, provided that the lesions were initially FDG-avid and no adjuvant chemotherapy is administered. Whenever this is the case, MR imaging is the modality of choice.

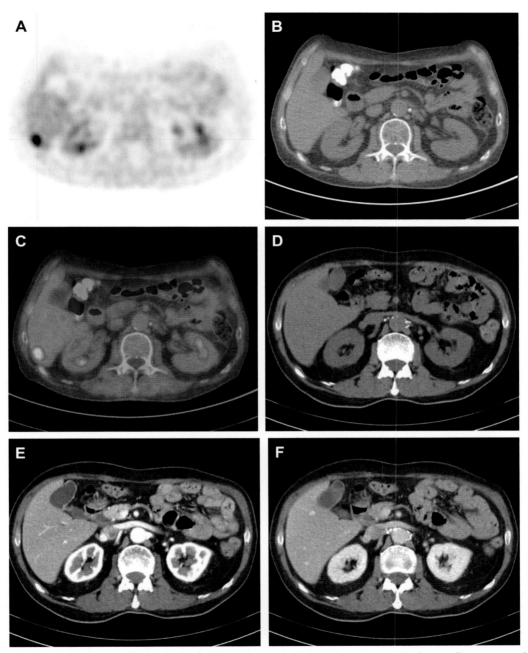

Fig. 2. A 75-year-old man is referred before surgical resection of a rectal cancer. PET/CT shows a liver metastasis in the segment of the liver (*A*, PET; *B*, low-dose, unenhanced CT; *C*, fused images). Diagnostic CT is negative (*D*, unenhanced; *E*, arterial phase; *F*, portal phase).

FDG-PET is also able to evaluate the metabolic response after intraarterial ^{90}Y-microsphere treatment of liver metastases.[4,43] However, only preliminary data are available and the technique requires further validation before it could be routinely proposed.

SUMMARY

FDG PET/CT has strongly established its high diagnostic accuracy for diagnosing liver metastases from colorectal cancers as well as from most malignant tumors. The vast majority of the patients are accurately staged with PET/CT, without the need for contrast-enhanced CT. PET/CT has limitations, especially for detecting very small lesions, which are better visualized with MR imaging, although the specificity of MR imaging may be an issue. The optimal preoperative liver staging probably combines MR imaging with PET/CT; in this case with IV contrast enhancement to precisely define the segmental localization of the lesions. PET/CT has a significant positive impact on the management of patients, thanks to a high accuracy both inside and outside the liver. The results are encouraging in patients treated with locoregional approaches, although further validation is needed.

REFERENCES

1. Bhattacharya R, Rao S, Kowdley KV. Liver involvement in patients with solid tumors of nonhepatic origin. Clin Liver Dis 2002;6(4):1033–43, x.
2. Pawlik TM, Schulick RD, Choti MA. Expanding criteria for resectability of colorectal liver metastases. Oncologist 2008;13(1):51–64.
3. Lim L, Gibbs P, Yip D, et al. A prospective evaluation of treatment with Selective Internal Radiation Therapy (SIR-spheres) in patients with unresectable liver metastases from colorectal cancer previously treated with 5-FU based chemotherapy. BMC Cancer 2005;5:132.
4. Lewandowski RJ, Thurston KG, Goin JE, et al. 90Y microsphere (TheraSphere) treatment for unresectable colorectal cancer metastases of the liver: response to treatment at targeted doses of 135-150 Gy as measured by [18F]fluorodeoxyglucose positron emission tomography and computed tomographic imaging. J Vasc Interv Radiol 2005;16(12):1641–51.
5. Kuvshinoff B, Fong Y. Surgical therapy of liver metastases. Semin Oncol 2007;34(3):177–85.
6. Choi J. Imaging of hepatic metastases. Cancer Control 2006;13(1):6–12.
7. Dietrich CF, Kratzer W, Strobe D, et al. Assessment of metastatic liver disease in patients with primary extrahepatic tumors by contrast-enhanced sonography versus CT and MRI. World J Gastroenterol 2006;12(11):1699–705.
8. Albrecht T, Blomley MJ, Burns PN, et al. Improved detection of hepatic metastases with pulse-inversion US during the liver-specific phase of SHU 508A: multicenter study. Radiology 2003;227(2):361–70.
9. Albrecht T, Hoffmann CW, Schmitz SA, et al. Phase-inversion sonography during the liver-specific late phase of contrast enhancement: improved detection of liver metastases. AJR Am J Roentgenol 2001;176(5):1191–8.
10. Soyer P, Poccard M, Boudiaf M, et al. Detection of hypovascular hepatic metastases at triple-phase helical CT: sensitivity of phases and comparison with surgical and histopathologic findings. Radiology 2004;231(2):413–20.
11. Sheafor DH, Frederick MG, Paulson EK, et al. Comparison of unenhanced, hepatic arterial-dominant, and portal venous-dominant phase helical CT for the detection of liver metastases in women with breast carcinoma. AJR Am J Roentgenol 1999;172(4):961–8.
12. van Erkel AR, Pijl ME, van den Berg-Huysmans AA, et al. Hepatic metastases in patients with colorectal cancer: relationship between size of metastases, standard of reference, and detection rates. Radiology 2002;224(2):404–9.
13. Kamel IR, Georgiades C, Fishman EK. Incremental value of advanced image processing of multislice computed tomography data in the evaluation of hypervascular liver lesions. J Comput Assist Tomogr 2003;27(4):652–6.
14. Rappeport ED, Loft A, Berthelsen AK, et al. Contrast-enhanced FDG-PET/CT vs. SPIO-enhanced MRI vs. FDG-PET vs. CT in patients with liver metastases from colorectal cancer: a prospective study with intraoperative confirmation. Acta Radiol 2007;48(4):369–78.
15. Namasivayam S, Martin DR, Saini S. Imaging of liver metastases: MRI. Cancer Imaging 2007;7:2–9.
16. Kim HJ, Kim KW, Byun JH, et al. Comparison of mangafodipir trisodium- and ferucarbotran-enhanced MRI for detection and characterization of hepatic metastases in colorectal cancer patients. AJR Am J Roentgenol 2006;186(4):1059–66.
17. Choi JY, Kim MJ, Kim JH, et al. Detection of hepatic metastasis: manganese- and ferucarbotran-enhanced MR imaging. Eur J Radiol 2006;60(1):84–90.
18. Bartolozzi C, Donati F, Cioni D, et al. Detection of colorectal liver metastases: a prospective multicenter trial comparing unenhanced MRI, MnDPDP-enhanced MRI, and spiral CT. Eur Radiol 2004;14(1):14–20.
19. Ward J, Robinson PJ, Guthrie JA, et al. Liver metastases in candidates for hepatic resection: comparison of helical CT and gadolinium- and SPIO-enhanced MR imaging. Radiology 2005;237(1):170–80.
20. Schima W, Kulinna C, Langenberger H, et al. Liver metastases of colorectal cancer: US, CT or MR? Cancer Imaging 2005;5(Spec No A):S149–56.
21. Yonekura Y, Benua RS, Brill AB, et al. Increased accumulation of 2-deoxy-2-[18F]Fluoro-D-glucose in liver metastases from colon carcinoma. J Nucl Med 1982;23(12):1133–7.
22. Delbeke D, Martin WH, Sandler MP, et al. Evaluation of benign vs malignant hepatic lesions with positron emission tomography. Arch Surg 1998;133(5):510–5 [discussion: 5–6].
23. Hustinx R, Paulus P, Jacquet N, et al. Clinical evaluation of whole-body 18F-fluorodeoxyglucose

positron emission tomography in the detection of liver metastases. Ann Oncol 1998;9(4):397–401.

24. Lai DT, Fulham M, Stephen MS, et al. The role of whole-body positron emission tomography with [18F]fluorodeoxyglucose in identifying operable colorectal cancer metastases to the liver. Arch Surg 1996;131(7):703–7.

25. Vitola JV, Delbeke D, Sandler MP, et al. Positron emission tomography to stage suspected metastatic colorectal carcinoma to the liver. Am J Surg 1996; 171(1):21–6.

26. Kinkel K, Lu Y, Both M, et al. Detection of hepatic metastases from cancers of the gastrointestinal tract by using noninvasive imaging methods (US, CT, MR imaging, PET): a meta-analysis. Radiology 2002; 224(3):748–56.

27. Bipat S, van Leeuwen MS, Comans EF, et al. Colorectal liver metastases: CT, MR imaging, and PET for diagnosis–meta-analysis. Radiology 2005; 237(1):123–31.

28. Wiering B, Krabbe PF, Jager GJ, et al. The impact of fluor-18-deoxyglucose-positron emission tomography in the management of colorectal liver metastases. Cancer 2005;104(12):2658–70.

29. Wiering B, Ruers TJ, Krabbe PF, et al. Comparison of multiphase CT, FDG-PET and intra-operative ultrasound in patients with colorectal liver metastases selected for surgery. Ann Surg Oncol 2007;14(2): 818–26.

30. Fernandez FG, Drebin JA, Linehan DC, et al. Five-year survival after resection of hepatic metastases from colorectal cancer in patients screened by positron emission tomography with F-18 fluorodeoxyglucose (FDG-PET). Ann Surg 2004;240(3):438–47 [discussion: 47–50].

31. Riedl CC, Akhurst T, Larson S, et al. 18F-FDG PET scanning correlates with tissue markers of poor prognosis and predicts mortality for patients after liver resection for colorectal metastases. J Nucl Med 2007;48(5):771–5.

32. Cohade C, Osman M, Leal J, et al. Direct comparison of (18)F-FDG PET and PET/CT in patients with colorectal carcinoma. J Nucl Med 2003;44(11): 1797–803.

33. Selzner M, Hany TF, Wildbrett P, et al. Does the novel PET/CT imaging modality impact on the treatment of patients with metastatic colorectal cancer of the liver? Ann Surg 2004;240(6):1027–34 [discussion: 35–6].

34. Lubezky N, Metser U, Geva R, et al. The role and limitations of 18-fluoro-2-deoxy-D-glucose positron emission tomography (FDG-PET) scan and computerized tomography (CT) in restaging patients with hepatic colorectal metastases following neoadjuvant chemotherapy: comparison with operative and pathological findings. J Gastrointest Surg 2007;11(4): 472–8.

35. Kong G, Jackson C, Koh DM, et al. The use of (18) F-FDG PET/CT in colorectal liver metastases—comparison with CT and liver MRI. Eur J Nucl Med Mol Imaging 2008;35(7):1323–9.

36. Chua SC, Groves AM, Kayani I, et al. The impact of 18F-FDG PET/CT in patients with liver metastases. Eur J Nucl Med Mol Imaging 2007;34(12):1906–14.

37. Soyka JD, Veit-Haibach P, Strobel K, et al. Staging pathways in recurrent colorectal carcinoma: is contrast-enhanced 18F-FDG PET/CT the diagnostic tool of choice? J Nucl Med 2008;49(3):354–61.

38. Kuehl H, Rosenbaum-Krumme S, Veit-Haibach P, et al. Impact of whole-body imaging on treatment decision to radio-frequency ablation in patients with malignant liver tumors: comparison of [18F]fluorodeoxyglucose-PET/computed tomography, PET and computed tomography. Nucl Med Commun 2008;29(7):599–606.

39. Veit P, Antoch G, Stergar H, et al. Detection of residual tumor after radiofrequency ablation of liver metastasis with dual-modality PET/CT: initial results. Eur Radiol 2006;16(1):80–7.

40. Anderson GS, Brinkmann F, Soulen MC, et al. FDG positron emission tomography in the surveillance of hepatic tumors treated with radiofrequency ablation. Clin Nucl Med 2003;28(3):192–7.

41. Travaini LL, Trifiro G, Ravasi L, et al. Role of [(18)F]FDG-PET/CT after radiofrequency ablation of liver metastases: preliminary results. Eur J Nucl Med Mol Imaging 2008;35(7):1316–22.

42. Kuehl H, Antoch G, Stergar H, et al. Comparison of FDG-PET, PET/CT and MRI for follow-up of colorectal liver metastases treated with radiofrequency ablation: initial results. Eur J Radiol 2008;67(2): 362–71.

43. Wong CY, Salem R, Qing F, et al. Metabolic response after intraarterial 90Y-glass microsphere treatment for colorectal liver metastases: comparison of quantitative and visual analyses by 18F-FDG PET. J Nucl Med 2004;45(11):1892–7.

PET/CT in Neuroendocrine Tumors

Paolo Castellucci, MD*, Valentina Ambrosini, MD, PhD,
Giancarlo Montini, MD

KEYWORDS

- Neuroendocrine tumors
- Positron emission tomography • Diagnosis

Neuroendocrine tumors (NETs) are a heterogeneous group of slow-growing rare neoplasms characterized by their endocrine metabolism and histology pattern, occurring in 1 to 4 per 100,000 people per year,[1,2] mostly represented by carcinoid lesions. These tumors originate from pluripotent stem cells or differentiated neuroendocrine cells.[3] Histologically, NETs can be classified on the basis of degree of differentiation in three classes: type 1a are well differentiated NETs (Ki-67 <2%), type 1b are well-differentiated neuroendocrine carcinomas (Ki-67 2%–10%), and type 2 are poorly differentiated neuroendocrine carcinomas.[4] NET cells belong to the amine precursor uptake and decarboxilation (APUD) cells system and can produce a large variety of substances because they take up, accumulate, and decarboxylate amine precursors, such as 3,4-dihydroxyl-phenylalanine (DOPA) and 5-hydroxytryptophan. Tumors deriving from these cells consequently were called APUDomas in the past. Another characteristic of these neoplasms is that they express several different peptide receptors in high quantities. These two characteristics are important for the diagnostic approach of molecular imaging of these tumors and are discussed elsewhere in this issue.

The most common sites of NET onset are the bronchus/lungs and gastroenteropancreatic tract. Less frequent localizations are the skin, adrenal glands, thyroid, and genital tract.[5] NETs can be functional or nonfunctional on the basis of the presence or absence of symptoms (related to NET hormones production). Approximately 33% to 50% of all the NETs are functional. The most important single prognostic factor for survival and prognosis is the presence of liver metastases: secondary lesions in the liver are present in approximately 15% to 25% of NETs if the tumor diameter is less than 1 cm, in 58% to 80% if it is 1 to 2 cm, and greater than 75% if the tumor size is greater than 2 cm.[5]

Finally, it is worth remembering that the diagnosis of primary NET lesions may be difficult because they often present as small lesions with variable anatomic locations. In the past few years, many different positron-emitter radiopharmaceuticals have been developed for the diagnosis of these rare tumors.

This article analyzes the results achieved PET in the assessment of NETs.

DIAGNOSIS OF NEUROENDOCRINE TUMORS

When NET is suspected, the first approach should be the analysis of laboratory data and the execution of conventional imaging (CI) procedures, such as CT, MR imaging, ultrasound (US), and endoscopic US. The second step should be, when possible, a biopsy to confirm the diagnosis.

Laboratory Data

Depending on the clinical suspicion of the presence of a NET, these different markers should be measured:

> Chromogranin A:changes in level over 25% are considered significant (conditions leading to elevated level of chromogranin A other than NET include hypergastrinemia,

Department of Nuclear Medicine, Policlinico S.Orsola-Malpighi, University of Bologna, Padiglione 30, Via Massarenti 9, 40138 Bologna, Italy
* Corresponding author.
E-mail address: paolo.castellucci@aosp.bo.it (P. Castellucci).

PET Clin 3 (2008) 197–205
doi:10.1016/j.cpet.2008.08.007

renal insufficiency, severe hypertension, and so forth).

Gastrin:fasting level should be measured in case a gastrinoma is suspected.

Insulin:for insulinoma, elevated level should be demonstrated in fasting condition.

Metanephrines or catecholamines:for pheochromocytoma, metanephrines, and catecholamines metabolites should be measured in the blood/urine.[5]

Histology

Recent World Health Organization classification[6] and new TNM staging take into account the different histopathologic behavior of NETs and were demonstrated to correlate well with the prognosis. NETs are classified as well-differentiated endocrine tumor, well-differentiated endocrine carcinoma, poorly differentiated endocrine carcinoma, mixed exocrine-endocrine tumor, and tumor-like lesions. NETs of the gastroenteropancreatic tract also can be classified depending on their origin in NET of the foregut (pancreas, stomach, or duodenum), midgut (ileum or appendix), or hindgut (colon or rectum).

Conventional Imaging

For many different reasons, CI techniques have poor accuracy in the diagnosis of NET and limited usefulness for patients' clinical management. A lack of sensitivity for CI (US, CT, and MR imaging) has been demonstrated by Gabriel and colleagues[7] mainly for detecting primary lesions in specific anatomic areas (such as small bowel) and in the detection of small bone and lymph node lesions. Moreover, as for many other tumors, the assessment of response to therapy is difficult according only to morphologic data.

Finally, in the field of NETs, CI techniques are not able to address patients to specific treatment, such as peptide radionuclide receptor therapy (PRRT). For all the reasons discussed previously, the diagnosis of NET is a field in which molecular imaging can provide significant, and sometimes unique, information for the most appropriate clinical management of these patients.

PET/CT-RADIOLABELED COMPOUNDS IN THE DIAGNOSIS OF NEUROENDOCRINE TUMORS

In the past decades, molecular imaging and, in particular, somatostatin receptor scintigraphy (SSR-S), has been used successfully for the assessment of patients who have NET. Nowadays, however, PET also is increasingly used for the detection of NETs, for the assessment of the

response to treatment, and for the selection of patient candidates for PRRT. This article reviews the role of different radiolabeled positron emission compounds for the study of patients who have NET.

Positron-emitter radiopharmaceuticals can be classified into two groups (**Table 1**) depending on the mechanism of uptake:

Receptor radiopharmaceuticals: several compounds binding somatostatin receptors, thus investigating the somatostatin receptor expression, belong to this group.

Metabolic radiopharmacuticals: includes PET tracers that allow investigating different metabolic pathways, such as serotonin production pathway, biogenic amine storage, catecholamine transport and glucose metabolism.

Receptor Radiopharmaceuticals: Positron-Emitter Radiopharmaceuticals Binding to Somatostatin Receptors

Several radiopharmaceuticals have been designed to specifically bind to somatostatin receptors (SSTRs) that are highly expressed on NET cells. Among the five different SSTRs, most of the NETs express SSTR2, with lower percentages of SSTR1 and SSTR5.[8–10] Several different somatostatin analogs (DOTA-TOC, DOTA-TATE, and DOTA-NOC) have been described for PET use[11] and they present differences in the binding affinity to SSTRs. Somatostatin-radiolabeled compounds (see **Table 1**) are derivatives of octreotide, lanreotide, or vapreotide and show variable binding to SSTRs.[12–14] DOTA-TOC, DOTA-TATE, and DOTA-NOC all bind to SSR2, the predominant receptor type in NET, and to SSR5, whereas only ^{68}Ga-DOTA-NOC also presents a good affinity for SSR3. One of the advantages of using such tracers for routine clinical use is that they can be labeled with ^{68}Ga, produced from a Ge-68/^{68}Ga generator. The synthesis and labeling process is easy and does not require an on-site cyclotron. [68]Ga ($t_{1/2}$ = 68 min) is a positron emitter with 89% positron emission and negligible gamma emission (1077 keV) of 3.2 % only. The long half-life of the mother radionuclide, [68]Ge (270.8 days), makes it possible to use the generator for approximately 9 to 12 months depending on the requirement. Rösch and Knapp[15] first described a method for a simple labeling procedure.[16] Radiolabeling yields of greater than 95% usually can be achieved within 15 minutes. Overall, 300 to 700 MBq of ^{68}Ga-DOTA-NOC are obtained within 20 minutes.

Table 1
Principal PET radiopharmaceuticals for the diagnosis of neuroendocrine tumors

Radiopharmaceutical	Target	Indication
^{68}Ga-DOTA-NOC	SSTRs Affinity for SSTRs 2,3,5	All SSTRs + NET
^{68}Ga-DOTA-TOC	SSTRs Affinity for SSTR2	All SSTRs + NET
[11]C-5-HTP	Serotonin production pathway	All serotonin-producing NETs
^{18}F-DOPA	Dopamine production pathway	Pheochromocytoma, paraganglioma, neuroblastoma, glomus tumor, medullary thyroid carcinoma, hyperinsulinism
^{18}F-FDA	Catecholamine precursor	Pheochromocytoma, paraganglioma, neuroblastoma
[11]C-ephidrine	Catecholamine transporter	Pheochromocytoma, neuroblastoma
[11]C-HED	Catecholoamine transporter	Pheochromocytoma, neuroblastoma
^{18}F-FDG	Glycolytic pathway	All poorly differentiated NETs

^{68}Ga-DOTA-TOC was the first radiopharmaceutical used for PET imaging of NET; however, Wild and colleagues[13,14] have shown that the compound ^{68}Ga-DOTA-NOC has 3 to 4 times higher binding affinity to SSTRs 2, 3, and 5, which results in coverage of a wide spectrum of SSTRs (pansomatostatin analog) and has significant effect on staging, diagnosis, and therapy of NETs and various other SSTR-expressing tumors.

Metabolic Radiopharmaceuticals

Radiopharmaceuticals targeting serotonin production pathway

Most of the clinical symptoms of a neuroendocrine tumor are the result of excessive production of serotonin. 5-Hydroxytryptophan is one of the intermediates in the production pathway and was successfully labeled with [11]C.[17,18] Unfortunately, the technical difficulties of labeling 5-hydroxytryptophan to ^{11}C make this compound difficult to produce extensively.

Radiopharmaceuticals targeting biogenic amine production and storage mechanism

Several biogenic amines are produced and stored by NETs. The use of fluorine-18 (^{18}F)-labeled L-DOPA (^{18}F-DOPA) is based on this observation. ^{18}F-DOPA is an aromatic amino acid labeled with ^{18}F that was first used in patients who had Parkinson's disease.[19] More recently, ^{18}F-DOPA has been used to differentiate between focal and diffuse congenital hyperglycemia[20] and to study NETs.[21] Belonging to the APUD cells system, NET cells are avid of ^{18}F-DOPA and, therefore, can be visualized on ^{18}F-DOPA PET scans.

^{18}F-DOPA is excreted trough the bile ducts, gallbladder, and digestive and urinary tracts.[21]

Radiopharmaceuticals targeting catecholamine transport pathway

Pheochromocytoma, neuroblastoma, and other chromaffin tissues concentrate many synthetic amine precursors and catecholamine, such as ^{11}C-epinephrine and ^{11}C-hydroxyephedrine (^{11}C-HED).

Radiopharmaceuticals targeting increased glucose metabolism

[18]F-2-fluoro-2-deoxyglucose (^{18}F-FDG) targets the glycolytic pathway, the main source of glucose consumption in tumors. ^{18}F-FDG enters the glycolytic pathway just like glucose and is phosphorylated by hexokinase to ^{18}F-FDG-6-phosphate. The fluorinated compound is not metabolized further and is trapped inside the cancer cell.

PET/CT IMAGING PROTOCOLS
Receptor PET/CT using ^{68}Ga-DOTA-peptides

PET/CT acquisition is started 60 minutes (30–180 min) after intravenous injection of approximately 100 MBq (75–250 MBq) of the radiolabeled peptide (such as ^{68}Ga-DOTA-NOC or DOTA-TOC). The amount of injected radioactivity depends on the daily production of the generator for each single elution (usually ranging between 300 and 700 MBq) and by the number of patients scanned per day.

The excretion of DOTA-peptides is primarily through the kidney, making it the critical organ.

Urinary bladder and spleen also receive high radiation doses; however, the overall radiation dose delivered to the other organs by ^{68}Ga-DOTA-NOC is comparable to, and even lower than, other diagnostic analogs, as reported by Pettinato and colleagues[22] in the first and only study published about the biodistribution of Ga-DOTA-NOC in nine patients who had NET. This evidence, in addition to the fact that DOTA-NOC covers the wider range of SSTRs, makes an interesting and positive observation.

Metabolic PET/CT Imaging Protocol

^{18}F-DOPA PET is performed after the intravenous injection of 5 to 6 MBq/kg, with an uptake time ranging from 60 to 90 minutes. Oral premedication with carbidopa, a peripheral aromatic amino acid decarboxylase inhibitor, was reported to enhance sensitivity by increasing the tumor-to-background ratio of tracer uptake.[22,23] Carbidopa administration, therefore, may be useful especially for the assessment of lesions at sites of increased ^{18}F-DOPA physiologic uptake, such as the pancreas.[24]

INDICATIONS FOR PET/CT

PET/CT, with ^{68}Ga-DOTA-NOC or metabolic radiopharmaceuticals, could play a role in staging, restaging, detection of unknown primary tumor, population selection for receptor-targeted therapies, and, finally, for the assessment of response to treatment. This section analyzes the usefulness of PET/CT in all these possible applications.

Staging and Re-Staging

Receptor PET/CT
NETs are difficult to diagnose without biopsy confirmation. The clinical symptoms are heterogeneous and the site of primary tumor may vary. Until now, ^{111}In-octreotide scintigraphy was considered the gold standard for NET diagnosis. Since 2001, few investigators compared the two imaging modalities (PET versus scintigraphy), reporting a better sensitivity of ^{68}Ga-DOTA-TOC PET/CT compared with ^{111}In-octreotide single photon emission CT (SPECT)[25,26] mainly for the detection of NET at lung, bone, and small lymph nodes levels. The main limitation of these studies, however, was the small populations studied. In April 2007, Gabriel and colleagues[7] reported the feasibility and high accuracy of ^{68}Ga-DOTA-TOC PET as a promising tool for the detection of NET in a large group of patients who had PET/CT for staging and restaging or for finding an occult primary cancer. On a patient basis, the accuracy of PET/CT (96%) was found significantly higher

than that of CT (75%) and ^{111}In-SSR-SPECT (58%). PET/CT was better than CT or SPECT as it detected more lesions in lymph nodes, liver, and bone. Overall, PET/CT provided clinically relevant information and was determinant to changing the clinical management in 14% of the patients when compared with SPECT and in 21% of patients when compared with CT.

Other studies confirmed these observations. Kowalski and colleagues[27] described that in comparison to the ^{111}In-SSR-SPECT, ^{68}Ga-DOTA-TOC PET/CT seems superior, especially in detecting small tumors or tumors bearing only a low density of SSTRs. Ambrosini and colleagues[28] recently compared ^{68}Ga-DOTA-NOC and ^{18}F-DOPA for the evaluation of gastroentero-pancreatic and lung NET in a small population (13 patients). ^{68}Ga-DOTA-NOC PET was positive, showing at least one lesion in all 13 cases whereas ^{18}F-DOPA PET was positive in only 9 of 13 patients. Moreover, on a lesions basis, ^{68}Ga-DOTA-NOC identified more lesions than ^{18}F-DOPA (71 versus 45), especially at liver, lung, and lymph nodes levels. The investigators concluded that, despite the limited and heterogeneous patient population, ^{68}Ga-DOTA-NOC was accurate for the detection of tumor in the primary or metastatic site and offered several advantages over ^{18}F-DOPA (**Fig. 1**).

Metabolic imaging
The use of ^{18}F-DOPA in the assessment of NETs has been investigated in the past few years. According to the conclusions of many studies, ^{18}F-DOPA seems superior to CI (US, CT, MR imaging, and SSR) with reported sensitivities ranging from 65% to 100%.[21,23,29–31] Koopmans compared ^{18}F-DOPA PET results with SSR and CT in 53 patients who had metastatic carcinoid tumor.[23] ^{18}F-DOPA PET presented a higher sensitivity than SSR and CT alone (100% versus 92% and 87%, respectively) or combined (96%). In their series, ^{18}F-DOPA was more sensitive, on a patient or on a lesion basis, than SSR and CT.

When compared with ^{68}Ga-DOTA-peptides, ^{18}F-DOPA may offer advantages for the detection of tumors with a low or absent expression of SSR, such as medullar thyroid carcinoma and undifferentiated NETs.[32,33]

In medullary thyroid cancer, a good sensitivity (63%) was reported for ^{18}F-DOPA PET with respect to other imaging procedures.[31] Only two studies in the literature, however, specifically in the role of ^{18}F-DOPA PET in patients who had medullary thyroid carcinoma. Moreover, the number of patients included in these studies was limited and in only a few cases ^{18}F-DOPA results could be confirmed by follow-up or pathology.[32,33] Therefore, further studies in larger series of patients are needed to assess the real usefulness of F-DOPA in patients who had medullary thyroid cancer.

Ambrosini and colleagues[34] also reported that in 13 patients who had biopsy-proved NET, ^{18}F-DOPA PET offered relevant information for the clinical management of patients who had an unclear clinical presentation or who had inconclusive findings at other imaging modalities (US, CT, SSR, or MR imaging). In particular, ^{18}F-DOPA PET changed patient management in 11 of 13 cases. Further surgery (other than that necessary to remove the primary tumor) was avoided in four cases, whereas in three patients, a metastatic surgical excision was guided by ^{18}F-DOPA PET/CT findings; in four nonoperable patients who had bone metastasis, chemotherapy was initiated after PET.

Pheocromocytoma is a condition in which CT, MR imaging, or ^{123}I-metaiodobenzylguanidine (MIBG) leaves up to 50% of malignant

lesions undetected. So the use of different radiopharmaceuticals has been proposed. In this clinical setting, ^{18}F-DOPA may offer advantages over ^{68}Ga-DOTA-peptides, because intact adrenal glands are a known site of ^{68}Ga-DOTA-peptides physiologic uptake, making them a difficult organ to explore. Two studies[30,35] reported how ^{18}F-DOPA PET can be particularly useful in these cases.

^{18}F-FDG PET is suggested for the diagnosis of undifferentiated and aggressive NET as reported by many investigators.[17,36–39] It was reported that ^{18}F-FDG PET was more sensitive than SSR (^{111}In-pentetreotide) for the detection of less differentiated gastroenteropancreatic tumors, whereas it was less sensitive for differentiated forms.

Finally, another clinically useful application of ^{18}F-DOPA is the distinction between focal and diffuse hyperinsulinism in pediatric patients, as reported by Ribeiro and colleagues.[20,40] In a recent publication, Barthlen and colleagues[41] confirmed the usefulness of ^{18}F-DOPA PET in 10 children who had focal congenital hyperinsulinism. All

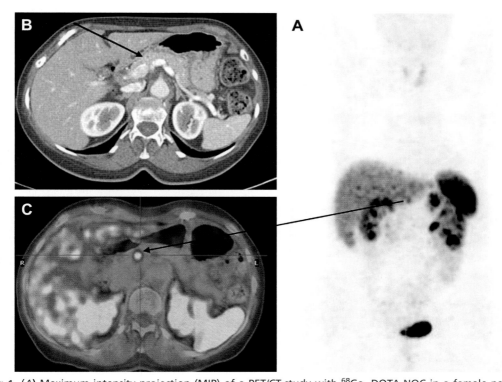

Fig. 1. (A) Maximum intensity projection (MIP) of a PET/CT study with ^{68}Ga-DOTA-NOC in a female patient (59 years old) who had hypoglycemia and suspected insulinoma. (B) Contrast-enhanced CT showed a small hypodense area in the head of the pancreas of unknown nature (black arrow). (C) Fusion images of the PET/CT study with ^{68}Ga-DOTA-NOC showed a small area of intense tracer uptake in the head of the pancreas (arrow). This finding is consistent with a primary insulinoma. Note the high tumor-to-background ratio. The lesion subsequently was removed surgically and histology confirmed the diagnosis of insulinoma.

patients were studied with ^{18}F-DOPA PET/CT before surgery. In 9 of 10 cases, intraoperative findings confirmed PET/CT presurgical findings. Hypoglycemia persisted in only one patient at follow-up, after two surgical resection of the pancreas.

In patients who had neuroblastoma ^{11}C-HED PET is particularly indicated, as reported by Shulkin and colleagues.[42,43] They compared the role of ^{123}I-MIBG and ^{11}C-HED PET and demonstrated that ^{11}C-HED PET presented a higher sensitivity. One of the limitations of ^{11}C-HED PET in this clinical setting was the high uptake in the liver, which interferes with liver lesion detection. Franzius and colleagues[44] confirmed the usefulness of ^{11}C-HED PET/CT in 19 patients who had neuroblastoma, pheocromocitoma, or paraganglioma in comparison with ^{123}I-MIBG. The high cost and the short half-life of ^{11}C, however, renders this radiolabeled compound difficult to use in daily practice.

Detection of Unknown Primary Tumor

Carcinoma of unknown primary tumor is defined as a biopsy-proved secondary lesion with no detectable primary tumor after physical examination and CI tests (chest radiograph, abdominal and pelvic CT, mammography in women, and so forth). This definition was proposed by Abbruzzese and colleagues,[45] who first analytically reviewed the diagnostic strategy of such a group of patients. The site of the occult primary tumor often remains unidentified after CI investigations in 20% to 27% of cases.[45,46]

Early identification of the primary tumor is a fundamental requisite for a prompt and targeted therapy and for changing patients' prognosis and

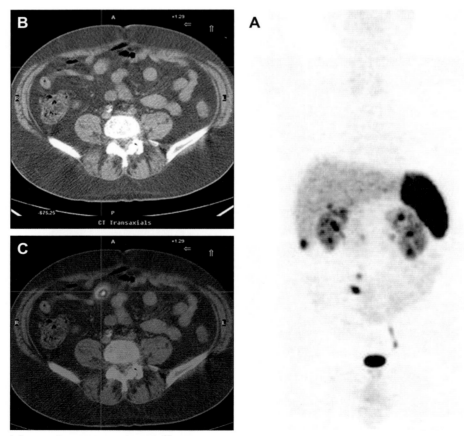

Fig. 2. (*A*) MIP of a PET/CT study with ^{68}Ga-DOTA-NOC in a male patient (62 years old) who had known liver metastasis and unknown site of the primary tumor. (*B*) Non–contrast-enhanced CT attenuation correction images. (*C*) Fusion images of the PET/CT study with ^{68}Ga-DOTA-NOC showed a small area of intense tracer uptake in a small bowel loop consistent with the primary site of a NET. The lesion subsequently was removed surgically and the histology confirmed the diagnosis of NET of the small bowel.

prolonging survival. This is true especially for NETs, because the unknown primary tumor in patients who have metastasis occurs more often than for other carcinomas. CT and MR imaging often fail to diagnose primary NET that (as discussed previously) can give clinical symptoms even when primary lesions are small in size.

In conclusion, PET/CT is a potentially useful tool for the detection of primary site of NET and for staging the extent of disease. Unfortunately, the recent wide application of PET/CT for the detection of NET of unknown primary origin provides no conclusive data regarding this issue, so no study has been addressed to assess the detection rate of PET/CT in NET of unknown primary tumor with receptor or metabolic PET/CT. This is a field, however, in which PET/CT theoretically is of great help. Hopefully in the near future a select patient population will be studied with PET/CT to confirm this hypothesis (**Fig. 2**).

Population Selection for Different Therapies

After correct diagnosis and accurate staging of NET, surgical resection and cold somatostatin analogs are used most commonly as first-line treatment. Recently, PRRT has been proposed as a highly effective treatment option for metastasized progressive NET. PRRT is considered more

and more as a third option for treatment protocol.[47] It is important to underline here that to initiate PRRT, ^{68}Ga-DOTA-NOC PET/CT is of extreme importance to document, in vivo, the expression of SSTRs on the tumor cells. The dose and the timing for PRRT (using [177]Lu- or ^{90}Y-DOTA-TOC) may depend on the semiquantitative and visual interpretation of the uptake of ^{68}Ga-DOTA-NOC measured by PET/CT.

As suggested by Ambrosini and colleagues,[28] patients' clinical management can be strongly influenced by ^{68}Ga-DOTA-NOC PET. The presence of a positive lesion on ^{68}Ga-DOTA-NOC reflects the presence of SSR on differentiated lesions that are more likely to respond to targeted therapy with cold somatostatin analogs or with PRRT.

^{68}Ga-DOTA-NOC providing additional data on receptor status, becoming a crucial pretherapy procedure, is a solid advantage of receptor PET/CT versus metabolic PET/CT in NET. Alternatively, a potential advantage of ^{18}F-DOPA (or other metabolic radiopharmaceuticals) over ^{68}Ga-DOTA-peptides may be represented by the more accurate evaluation of lesions with a low expression of SSTRs, such as poorly differentiated tumors and medullary thyroid carcinoma.

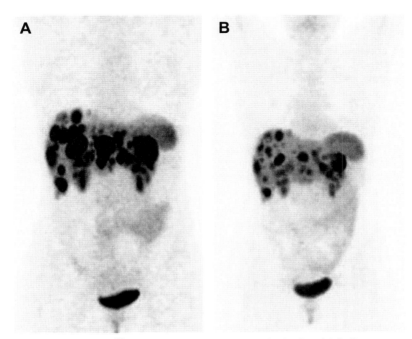

A   **B**

Fig. 3. (*A*) MIP of a PET/CT study with ^{68}Ga-DOTA-NOC in a patient who had multiple liver metastasis from NET of the pancreas. (*B*) MIP of a PET/CT study with ^{68}Ga-DOTA-NOC after three cycles of PRRT with ^{90}Y-DOTA-TOC. The treatment achieved a partial response.

Evaluation of Therapy Response

In the past few years ^{18}F-FDG PET/CT has been used successfully for therapy monitoring of many different cancers. The role of metabolic or receptor PET/CT, however, in the assessment of response to therapy in patients who have NET remains to be established. Receptor and metabolic PET/CT have the potential to correctly assess therapy response to cold or labeled somatostatin analogs or to chemotherapy, as for other cancers (**Fig. 3**). Currently, however, no study has been aimed specifically at assessing this potential role of PET/CT in a selected patient population.

SUMMARY

It can be concluded that ^{68}Ga-DOTA-peptides PET/CT probably will be applied more and more in patients who have NET in staging, restaging, or selection of patient candidates for PRRT. In particular, ^{68}GaDOTA-NOC PET/CT seems to provide superior information in comparison with conventional octreotide scintigraphy. The recent introduction on the market of low-cost Ge/Ga generators will make ^{68}Ga available even in PET centers that are not provided with a cyclotron. This will ensure that ^{68}Ga-DOTA-NOC PET/CT could be used in larger patient populations so that more accurate data on the effective impact on clinical management will be available.

In the field of metabolic PET/CT, ^{18}F-FDG PET/CT should be used in poorly differentiated NETs. Finally, F-DOPA and other radiopharmaceuticals seem to be useful and accurate in specific pathologic conditions, such as distinguishing between focal and diffuse hyperinsulinism, pheocromocytoma, neuroblastoma, and medullary thyroid cancer.

In conclusion, the wide spectrum of NETs that can have different clinical behavior and histologic characteristics requires a personalized diagnostic approach. PET/CT, with so many different radiopharmaceutical probes, can help clinicians in more accurate diagnosis and, therefore, better personalized therapeutic options.

REFERENCES

1. Modlin IM, Kidd M, Latich I, et al. Current status of gastrointestinal carcinoids. Gastroenterology 2005;128(6):1717–51.
2. Taal BG, Visser O. Epidemiology of neuroendocrine tumours. Neuroendocrinology 2004;80(Suppl 1):3–7.
3. Vinik AI, Woltering EA, O'Dorisio TM, et al. Neuroendocrine tumors: a comprehensive guide to diagnosis and management. Inter Science Institute; 2006.
4. Solcia E, Kloppel G, Sobin LH. Histological typing of tumors. In: Organisation WHOPPWH, editor. International histological classification of tumors in collaboration with 9 pathologists from 4 countries. 2nd edition. New York: Springer, Berlin Heidelberg; 2000.
5. Jensen RT. Endocrine tumors of the gastrointestinal tract and pancreas. In: Kasper DL, Fauci AS, Longo DL, editors. Harrison's principles of internal medicine. 16th edition. McGraw-Hill; 2005.
6. Rindi G, Kloppel G, Alhman H, et al. TNM staging of foregut (neuro)endocrine tumors: a consensus proposal including a grading system. Virchows Arch 2006;449:395.
7. Gabriel M, Decristoforo C, Kendler D, et al. ^{68}Ga-DOTA-Tyr3-octreotide PET in neuroendocrine tumors: comparison with somatostatin receptor scintigraphy and CT. J Nucl Med 2007;48:508.
8. Reubi JC. Peptide receptors as molecular targets for cancer diagnosis and therapy. Endocr Rev 2003;24:389.
9. Reubi JC, Schar JC, Waser B, et al. Affinity profiles for human somatostatin receptor subtypes SST1-SST5 of somatostatin radiotracers selected for scintigraphic and radiotherapeutic use. Eur J Nucl Med 2000;27:273.
10. Reubi JC, Waser B, Schaer JC, et al. Somatostatin receptor sst1-sst5 expression in normal and neoplastic human tissues using receptor autoradiography with subtype-selective ligands. Eur J Nucl Med 2001;28:836.
11. Antunes P, Ginj M, Zhang H, et al. Are radiogallium-labeled DOTA-conjugated somatostatin analogues superior to those labeled with other radiometals? Eur J Nucl Med Mol Imaging 2007;34(7):982–3.
12. Rufini V, Calcagni ML, Baum RP. Imaging of neuroendocrine tumors. Semin Nucl Med 2006;36:228.
13. Wild D, Macke HR, Waser B, et al. ^{68}Ga-DOTANOC: a first compound for PET imaging with high affinity for somatostatin receptor subtypes 2 and 5. Eur J Nucl Med Mol Imaging 2005;32:724.
14. Wild D, Schmitt JS, Ginj M, et al. DOTA-NOC, a high-affinity ligand of somatostatin receptor subtypes 2, 3 and 5 for labeling with various radiometals. Eur J Nucl Med Mol Imaging 2003;30:1338.
15. Rösch F, Knapp FFRIn: Radionuclide generators, vol 4. Rotterdam (NL): Kluwer Academic Publishers; 2003.
16. Zhernosekov KP, Filosofov DV, Baum RP, et al. Processing of generator-produced ^{68}Ga for medical application. J Nucl Med 2007;48:1741.
17. Eriksson B, Bergstrom M, Orlefors H, et al. Use of PET in neuroendocrine tumors. In vivo applications and in vitro studies. Q J Nucl Med 2000;44:68.
18. Orlefors H, Sundin A, Ahlstrom H, et al. Positron emission tomography with 5-hydroxytryprophan in neuroendocrine tumors. J Clin Oncol 1998;16:2534.
19. Eidelberg D, Moeller JR, Dhawan V, et al. The metabolic anatomy of Parkinson's disease: complementary [18F]fluorodeoxyglucose and

[18F]fluorodopa positron emission tomographic studies. Mov Disord 1990;5:203.

20. Ribeiro MJ, Boddaert N, Bellanne-Chantelot C, et al. The added value of [(18)F]fluoro-L: -DOPA PET in the diagnosis of hyperinsulinism of infancy: a retrospective study involving 49 children. Eur J Nucl Med Mol Imaging 2007;34:2120.

21. Hoegerle S, Altehoefer C, Ghanem N, et al. Whole-body 18F dopa PET for detection of gastrointestinal carcinoid tumors. Radiology 2001;220:373.

22. Pettinato C, Sarnelli A, Di Donna M. (68)Ga-DOTA-NOC: biodistribution and dosimetry in patients affected by neuroendocrine tomors. Eur J Nucl Med Mol Imaging 2008;35(1):72–9.

23. Koopmans KP, de Vries EG, Kema IP, et al. Staging of carcinoid tumours with 18F-DOPA PET: a prospective, diagnostic accuracy study. Lancet Oncol 2006; 7:728.

24. Timmers HJ, Hadi M, Carrasquillo JA, et al. The effects of carbidopa on uptake of 6-18F-Fluoro-L-DOPA in PET of pheochromocytoma and extraadrenal abdominal paraganglioma. J Nucl Med 2007;48:1599.

25. Buchmann I, Henze M, Engelbrecht S, et al. Comparison of 68Ga-DOTATOC PET and 111In-DTPAOC (Octreoscan) SPECT in patients with neuroendocrine tumours. Eur J Nucl Med Mol Imaging 2007; 34:1617.

26. Hofmann M, Maecke H, Borner R, et al. Biokinetics and imaging with the somatostatin receptor PET radioligand (68)Ga-DOTATOC: preliminary data. Eur J Nucl Med 2001;28:1751.

27. Kowalski J, Henze M, Schuhmacher J, et al. Evaluation of positron emission tomography imaging using [68Ga]-DOTA-D Phe(1)-Tyr(3)-Octreotide in comparison to [111In]-DTPAOC SPECT. First results in patients with neuroendocrine tumors. Mol Imaging Biol 2003;5:42.

28. Ambrosini V, Tomassetti P. Castellucci P comparison between 68Ga-DOTA-NOC and 18F-DOPA PET for the detection of gastro-entero-pancreatic and lung neuroendocrine tumours. Eur J Nucl Med Mol Imaging. 2008 April, 17 [Epub ahead of print].

29. Becherer A, Szabo M, Karanikas G, et al. Imaging of advanced neuroendocrine tumors with (18)F-FDOPA PET. J Nucl Med 2004;45:1161.

30. Hoegerle S, Nitzsche E, Altehoefer C, et al. Pheochromocytomas: detection with 18F DOPA whole body PET–initial results. Radiology 2002;222:507.

31. Nanni C, Fanti S, Rubello D. 18F-DOPA PET and PET/CT. J Nucl Med 2007;48:1577.

32. Beuthien-Baumann B, Strumpf A, Zessin J, et al. Diagnostic impact of PET with 18F-FDG, 18F-DOPA and 3-O-methyl-6-[18F]fluoro-DOPA in recurrent or metastatic medullary thyroid carcinoma. Eur J Nucl Med Mol Imaging 2007;34:1604.

33. Hoegerle S, Altehoefer C, Ghanem N, et al. 18F-DOPA positron emission tomography for tumour detection in patients with medullary thyroid carcinoma and elevated calcitonin levels. Eur J Nucl Med 2001;28:64.

34. Ambrosini V, Tomassetti P, Rubello D, et al. Role of 18F-dopa PET/CT imaging in the management of patients with 111In-pentetreotide negative GEP tumours. Nucl Med Commun 2007;28:473.

35. Mackenzie IS, Gurnell M, Balan KK, et al. The use of 18-fluoro-dihydroxyphenylalanine and 18-fluoro-deoxyglucose positron emission tomography scanning in the assessment of metaiodobenzylguanidine-negative phaeochromocytoma. Eur J Endocrinol 2007;157:533.

36. Pasquali C, Rubello D, Sperti C, et al. Neuroendocrine tumor imaging: can 18F-fluorodeoxyglucose positron emission tomography detect tumors with poor prognosis and aggressive behavior? World J Surg 1998;22:588.

37. Scanga DR, Martin WH, Delbeke D. Value of FDG PET imaging in the management of patients with thyroid, neuroendocrine, and neural crest tumors. Clin Nucl Med 2004;29:86.

38. Sundin A, Eriksson B, Bergstrom M, et al. PET in the diagnosis of neuroendocrine tumors. Ann N Y Acad Sci 2004;1014:246.

39. Zhao DS, Valdivia AY, Li Y, et al. 18F-fluorodeoxyglucose positron emission tomography in small-cell lung cancer. Semin Nucl Med 2002;32:272.

40. Ribeiro MJ, Boddaert N, Delsescauz T. Functional imaging of the pancreas: the role of 18F-DOPA PET in the diagnosis of hyperinsulinism of infancy. Endocr Dev 2007;12:55–66.

41. Barthlen W, Blankenstein O. Mau H evaluation of 18FDOPA PET/CT for surgery in focal congenital hyperinsulinism. J Clin Endocrinol Metab. 2008; 93(3):869–75.

42. Shulkin BL, Wieland DM, Baro ME, et al. PET hydroxyephedrine imaging of neuroblastoma. J Nucl Med 1996;37:16.

43. Shulkin BL, Wieland DM, Schwaiger M, et al. PET scanning with hydroxyephedrine: an approach to the localization of pheochromocytoma. J Nucl Med 1992;33:1125.

44. Franzius C, Hermann K, Weckesser M. Whole body PET/CT with 11C HED in tumors of the sympatetic nervous system: feasibility study and comparison with 123I MIBG SPECT /CT. J Nuc Med 2006;47(10):1635–42.

45. Abbruzzese JL, Abbruzzese MC, Lenzi R, et al. Analysis of a diagnostic strategy for patients with suspected tumors of unknown origin. J Clin Oncol 1995;13:2094.

46. Le Chevalier T, Cvitkovic E, Caille P, et al. Early metastatic cancer of unknown primary origin at presentation. A clinical study of 302 consecutive autopsied patients. Arch Intern Med 1988;148:2035.

47. Bodei L, Paganelli G. Receptor radionuclide therapy of tumors: a road from basic research to clinical application. J Nuc Med 2006;47(3):375–7.

Infrequent Tumors of the Gastrointestinal Tract Including Gastrointestinal Stromal Tumor (GIST)

Mehmet Ertuk, MD[a], Annick D. Van den Abbeele, MD[b,c,d,e],*

KEYWORDS

- Positron emission tomography • F-18-fluorodeoxyglucose
- Computed tomography • Gastrointestinal stromal tumor
- Imatinib • Sunitinib • Gastric lymphoma
- Intrapapillary mucinous neoplasm of the pancreas
- Gallbladder cancer

Although some tumors of the gastrointestinal system, such as gastrointestinal stromal tumor (GIST), gallbladder carcinoma, gastric lymphoma, and intrapapillary mucinous neoplasm of the pancreas, may not be encountered as frequently as others, the oncogenic signaling in these tumors is expected to drive glucose uptake as it does in more common tumors.[1] This addiction to sugar has been known since the 1930s, when Warburg[2] reported that cancer cells preferentially use glycolysis instead of oxidative phosphorylation in the presence of oxygen. This high rate of glycolysis exhibited by most tumors is required to support cell growth.[3] These principles support the use of the glucose analogue ^{18}F-fluorodeoxyglucose and positron emission tomography (FDG-PET) in most cancers including rare tumors.

There is now a hybrid system available which combines the anatomic information provided by CT with the functional evaluation provided by FDG-PET in one setting (FDG-PET/CT). Both FDG-PET and FDG-PET/CT have become indispensable tools in the management of patients with various cancers, including cancers of the gastrointestinal tract. The use of these imaging modalities has been well demonstrated in the staging of these cancers, restaging in the context of increased tumor markers, evaluation of surgical eligibility, and assessment of recurrence or residual disease. FDG-PET and FDG-PET/CT are now playing an increasing role in the evaluation of response to treatment. One of the best illustrations of the power of FDG-PET in the assessment of therapeutic response is in gastrointestinal stromal tumor (GIST), a rare tumor of the gastrointestinal tract, while testing two novel "tailored" therapies designed to match the tumor's genetic characteristics, ie, imatinib mesylate and sunitinib malate.

GASTROINTESTINAL STROMAL TUMORS

In 1983, Mazur and coworkers[4] described GIST as a subgroup of gastrointestinal mesenchymal tumors that are not classified as neurogenic- or smooth muscle-derived. Kindblom and colleagues[5] hypothesized that GIST may originate from the interstitial cell of Cajal in the normal myenteric plexus, an intestinal pacemaker cell.

[a] Department of Radiology, Şişli Etfal Training and Research Hospital, Şişli 34360, Istanbul, Turkey
[b] Department of Radiology, Dana-Farber Cancer Institute, 44 Binney Street, Boston, MA 02115, USA
[c] Harvard Medical School, Boston, MA, USA
[d] Center for Biomedical Imaging in Oncology, Dana-Farber Cancer Institute, 44 Binney Street, Boston, MA, USA
[e] Tumor Imaging Metrics Core, Dana-Farber/Harvard Cancer Center, 44 Binney Street, Boston, MA, USA
* Corresponding author.
E-mail address: abbeele@dfci.harvard.edu (A.D. Van den Abbeele).

PET Clin 3 (2008) 207–215
doi:10.1016/j.cpet.2008.10.002
1556-8598/08/$ – see front matter © 2008 Elsevier Inc. All rights reserved.

This hypothesis was confirmed by Hirota and co-workers[6] in 2000, who demonstrated that neoplastic GIST cells show ultrastructural features and express cell markers typical of the normal interstitial cell of Cajal.[7] On the basis of these developments, most gastrointestinal mesenchymal tumors previously designated as "smooth muscle tumors," such as leiomyomas, leiomyoblastomas, and leiomyosarcomas, are reclassified as GIST today.[7]

Although GIST is a rare tumor and accounts only for 0.1% to 3% of all gastrointestinal cancers, it is the most common kind of mesenchymal neoplasm of the alimentary tract,[8] and up to 20% of small bowel malignancies are GIST.[9] Primary GISTs are usually solitary tumors, and throughout the whole length of the gastrointestinal tract, GISTs arise most commonly in the stomach (60%–70%) followed by small bowel (20%–25%), and rarely from the rectum (5%), esophagus, colon, and appendix.[10]

GISTs are generally thought to be malignant, but they have different degrees of aggressiveness, resulting in varying times to the development of metastases.[11] At first diagnosis, approximately 10% of patients have metastatic disease,[10] but this incidence may actually be an underestimation because DeMatteo[12] reported that metastatic disease was found in nearly half of their patients. The liver is the most common site (65%) of metastatic disease, followed by the peritoneum (21%), whereas metastases to lymph nodes, bone, and lung are rare. Most patients develop recurrent GIST after an apparently complete surgical resection of the primary lesion. The common sites of recurrence are the liver, peritoneum, or both.[12]

The unique feature of GIST is that approximately 95% of these tumors are positive for KIT (CD117), the c-kit receptor tyrosine kinase.[13] In most GISTs, an activating mutation of c-kit leads to ligand-independent receptor dimerization and activation of KIT tyrosine kinase that promotes tumor survival and tumor growth.[14] More than 80% of GIST have an oncogenic mutation in the KIT tyrosine kinase,[15] and most of the mutations are in the juxtamembrane domain encoded by exon 11, but mutations may also occur in exons 9, 13, 17, PDGFRA.[16–18]

GISTs are known to be both chemoresistant and insensitive to irradiation, and surgical resection is the initial therapy for patients with primary GIST who have no metastases and are considered resectable. In the past, the lack of therapeutic options in inoperable and metastatic disease resulted in a generally poor prognosis in patients with GIST. Recent studies, however, have showed excellent results and greatly improved survival when GIST patients were treated with a new line of therapy using a selective small molecule that inhibits tumor growth by competitive interaction at the adenosine triphosphate binding site of the c-kit receptor (imatinib mesylate). Patients who have an exon 11 mutation within their tumors show the best response to imatinib therapy with an 85% response rate. There is also some suggestion that patients with exon 9 mutations may be more sensitive to sunitinib,[19] the second drug approved for treatment of GIST. Sunitinib also acts on VEGFR1-3, FLT-3, and RET adding a potential antiangiogenic effect. It is available to patients who are unresectable and have developed primary or secondary resistance to imatinib, and who are progressing despite higher doses of imatinib.[20]

As for the other intra-abdominal malignancies, CT scan is the standard preoperative imaging technique.[7] CT scan may reliably localize GIST, and determine size and possibly reveal the presence of secondary sites (eg, hepatic metastases).[7] Because most GISTs are FDG-avid, FDG-PET might be particularly useful in staging GIST patients to assess the extent of disease, but it has been mainly used for assessment of therapeutic response and patient follow-up.[7] As opposed to conventional cytotoxic chemotherapy where a decrease in the size of a tumor mass reflects response to therapy, reduction of viable tumor cells after therapy with tyrosine kinase inhibitors may not immediately result in a decrease in the tumor volume. In the case of imatinib and other molecular-targeted drugs, it might actually take weeks to months, even years, for tumors to shrink despite the fact that the patient is responding to the treatment. For optimal clinical outcome and to avoid unnecessary and costly treatment, the effect of imatinib on GIST needs to be defined soon after the start of therapy. Early detection of tumor response ensures effective therapy, while lack of response or progression requires a change in patient management.

The early evidence of biologic response by FDG-PET, and the insensitivity of morphologic response criteria, was first reported by the authors' group in 2001[21] (Fig. 1) and since confirmed by many research groups.[22–29] The results of subsequent clinical studies have strongly supported this observation. In the study of Jager and van der Graaf,[30] for example, 16 consecutive patients with unresectable or metastasized GIST or another c-kit (CD117) positive mesenchymal tumor underwent FDG-PET before and 1 week after the start of treatment with imatinib mesylate. In this study, FDG-PET visualized all known and some unknown tumor locations. The separation by FDG-PET after 1 week of treatment in PET responders (11 of 16

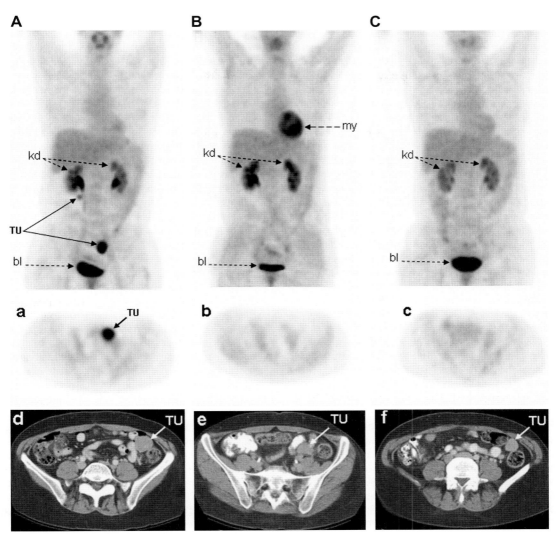

Fig. 1. FDG-PET maximum intensity projection images (A–C), axial PET (a–c), and axial CT (d–f) slices through the pelvis in a patient with metastatic GIST. Normal physiologic FDG uptake is seen (*dashed arrows*) in the urinary collecting system in both kidneys (kd), the myocardium (my), and in the bladder (bl). (*A*) Intense FDG uptake is seen in the left lower pelvis and contiguous to the right proximal ureter (TU, *straight arrows*) at baseline before imatinib therapy consistent with metastatic GIST. (*B*) Resolution of abnormal FDG uptake is noted in both tumor masses as early as 1 week following treatment with imatinib. (*C*) Continuous metabolic response to imatinib is seen in this patient 2 months following initiation of therapy despite the presence of a residual mass on CT. Axial FDG-PET slices obtained through the pelvis at the same time points (*a–c*) and correlative axial CT slices showing a FDG-avid mass in the left pelvis (TU, *black arrow*) before treatment (*a*), and resolution of abnormal FDG uptake on subsequent scans (*b, c*) despite a persistent mass on CT (TU, *white arrows*). TU, tumor.

patients, mean standardized uptake value [SUV] reduction of 65%) versus PET nonresponders (5 of 16 patients, mean SUV increase of 16%) seemed to match almost perfectly with overall treatment response and proved to be correct in 14 of 15 patients (prediction sensitivity, 93%). FDG uptake changes after 1 week of treatment were of greater magnitude than tumor volume changes on CT at 8 weeks. Progression-free survival was significantly better in patients with a PET response ($P = 0.002$). More importantly, PET response predicted treatment outcome better than the radiologic response.

Goerres and colleagues[31] have reported the prognostic power of FDG-PET, contrast-enhanced CT, and FDG-PET/CT in evaluating the therapeutic impact of treatment by imatinib mesylate in 34 patients with GIST. In 28 patients, FDG-PET/CT and contrast-enhanced CT were available after introduction of treatment with imatinib mesylate. Patients without FDG uptake after the start of treatment had a better prognosis than patients who showed residual activity. In comparison, contrast-enhanced CT criteria provided insufficient prognostic power. FDG-PET/CT delineated active lesions better than did the combination of FDG-PET and contrast-enhanced CT imaging. The authors concluded that both FDG-PET and FDG-PET/CT provided important prognostic information and that both have a significant impact on clinical decision-making in GIST patients.

Adding CT to FDG-PET increases the diagnostic accuracy. Antoch and colleagues[32] examined 20 patients with historically-proved GIST with FDG-PET/CT before, and 1, 3, and 6 months after the start of imatinib therapy. Separate FDG-PET and CT datasets, side-by-side FDG-PET and CT datasets, and fused FDG-PET/CT images were evaluated according to World Health Organization (WHO), Response Evaluation Criteria in Solid Tumors (RECIST), and European Organisation for Research and Treatment of Cancer (EORTC) criteria for therapeutic response. Hounsfield units (HU) were assessed on CT images. The numbers of lesions detected in all patients were 135 with FDG-PET, 249 with CT, 279 on side-by-side evaluation, and 282 on fused FDG-PET/CT images. Tumor response was correctly characterized in 95% of patients after 1 month, and 100% after 3 and 6 months with FDG-PET/CT. FDG-PET and CT images viewed side by side were correct in 90% of patients at 1 month, and 100% at 3 and 6 months. FDG-PET accurately diagnosed tumor response in 85% of patients at 1 month, and 100% at 3 and 6 months. CT was found to be accurate in 44% of patients at 1 month, 60% at 3 months, and 57% at 6 months. HU units were found to decrease by at least 25% in 12 of 14 responders after 1 month. The authors concluded that tumor response to imatinib should be assessed with a combination of morphologic and functional imaging. Image fusion with combined FDG-PET/CT can provide additional information in individual cases when compared with side-by-side FDG-PET and CT.

In a recent study from the authors' institution, Holdsworth and colleagues[33] aimed at optimizing the use of CT bidimensional measurements and FDG-PET maximum SUV (SUVmax) for determining response to imatinib mesylate treatment in patients with advanced GISTs. Sixty-three patients enrolled in the first multicenter trial evaluating imatinib mesylate therapy for advanced GIST underwent FDG-PET at baseline and 1 month after initiation of treatment. Of these 63 patients, 58 underwent concomitant CT. Time-to-treatment failure was used as the outcome measure. Patients were followed over a range of 23.7 to 37 months (median, 31.7 months). The predictive power of change in CT bidimensional measurements, change in FDG-PET SUVmax, and FDG-PET SUVmax at 1 month after initiation of treatment were determined, optimized, and compared. The effectiveness of combining metrics was also evaluated. The results showed that both a threshold FDG-PET SUVmax value of 2.5 at 1 month ($P = .04$) and the EORTC criteria for partial response on FDG-PET (25% reduction in SUVmax) at 1 month were predictive of prolonged treatment success ($P = .55$). The Southwest Oncology Group (SWOG) criteria for partial response (ie, 50% reduction in CT bidimensional measurements) at 1 month were not predictive of time-to-treatment failure ($P = .55$).

Another interesting observation was made on FDG-PET at the time of secondary resistance in patients receiving imatinib. These patients show increased FDG uptake at the tumor site (ie, a rebound phenomenon) following cessation of imatinib. When this was first observed, and disease recurrence was confirmed, these patients became eligible for enrollment in the trial that was then testing the second generation of tyrosine kinase inhibitors (sunitinib malate). Eligible patients were asked to stop imatinib before the start of sunitinib therapy, and a repeat FDG-PET was performed as the new baseline for the sunitinib trial. A significant rebound in glycolytic activity throughout the entire tumor mass was noted in patients who underwent two FDG-PET scans within 3 weeks or less between the end of imatinib therapy and before the initiation of sunitinib.[34] This rebound phenomenon suggests that part of the mass is still responding to imatinib, and that cessation of the drug leads to reactivation of glycolytic metabolism in tumor cells that are still responding to imatinib. The clonal differentiation that leads to secondary resistance and re-emergence of glycolytic activity probably affects another subpopulation of cells within that same tumor that has become resistant to the drug probably because of new mutational changes. This observation also suggests that compliance with the therapeutic regimen is important in order to keep the tumor metabolism at bay, and that combination therapy with more than one tyrosine kinase inhibitor might need to be studied in the future.

GALLBLADDER CANCER

Gallbladder cancer is a relatively rare disease. Surgical resection is the only therapeutic tool.[35]

Because gallbladder cancer has no specific symptoms, however, it is often diagnosed in advanced stages, and the 5-year survival rate for inoperable patients is below 10%, with a mean duration of survival of 6 months.[36,37] Furthermore it is also extremely difficult to detect gallbladder cancer in the early stage with conventional imaging modalities.[37] Although protuberant lesions can be detected and correctly characterized (malignant or benign) with conventional imaging modalities including ultrasound, CT, and MR imaging, cancers that manifest as gallbladder wall thickening remains a diagnostic dilemma because wall thickening is an imaging sign that is frequently encountered in the context of benign conditions, such as cholecystitis or adenomyomatosis.

There are some reports indicating that FDG-PET might be useful in the diagnosis of gallbladder cancer. Rodriguez-Frenandez and colleagues[38] reported that FDG-PET had a sensitivity of 75% and a specificity of 82% in a study of 16 cases of gallbladder disease (with gallbladder wall thickening observed in seven cases). In the study of Anderson and colleagues,[39] the authors evaluated the usefulness of FDG-PET in cases of gallbladder carcinoma and cholangiocarcinoma, and in 14 cases of gallbladder disease, and reported that the sensitivity of FDG-PET in detecting gallbladder cancer was 78%. In the study of Oe and colleagues,[36] when used to distinguish between malignant and benign gallbladder wall thickening, FDG-PET had a sensitivity of 75% and a specificity of 100%. In this study, of the 12 patients, 4 showed FDG uptake in the gallbladder wall. Of these four patients, three had gallbladder cancer and one had chronic cholecystitis and a false-positive finding. The other eight patients had negative uptake of FDG in the gallbladder wall. Two of these patients underwent surgical resection, which yielded a diagnosis of chronic cholecystitis. The other six patients exhibited no sign of gallbladder malignancy and have been followed without active treatment. It should be noted that both acute and chronic cholecystitis and xanthogranulomatous cholecystitis are reported to be sometimes falsely positive in the gallbladder wall thickening type[36] because FDG uptake can be seen within activated inflammatory cells.

PRIMARY GASTRIC LYMPHOMA

The incidence of non-Hodgkin's lymphoma (NHL) and, in particular, of extranodal lymphoma has increased over the last decades.[40] Primary gastric lymphoma is defined as an entity based on the presence of the bulk of disease in the stomach and a predominance of gastric and abdominal symptoms.[41,42] Although primary gastric lymphoma accounts for less than 5% of gastric neoplasms, it is one of the most common sites of extranodal lymphoma occurring in 4% to 20% of patients.[40–42] Clinical presentation and radiologic features of primary gastric lymphoma are in general nonspecific. Diagnosis is achieved mainly by endoscopy with biopsy. Histologically, primary gastric lymphoma is predominantly NHL, either high-grade, diffuse large B-cell lymphoma, or low-grade mucosa-associated lymphoid tissue, also defined in the World Health Organization classification as extranodal marginal zone B-cell lymphoma.[42,43]

Although there is strong scientific evidence supporting the use of FDG-PET in the initial evaluation and follow-up of patients with lymphoma,[44–47] the literature is sparse regarding the use of FDG-PET in patients with gastrointestinal tract lymphoma, and specifically primary gastric lymphoma.[40] The existing studies have controversial results in part because of the low or lack of FDG avidity of some histologic subtypes of the disease[40,48,49] and the presence of physiologic tracer uptake in the stomach. Nevertheless, combining the metabolic data obtained with FDG-PET with the anatomic data obtained with CT has the potential to improve the accuracy of detection and staging of gastric lymphoma.[50,51] FDG-PET/CT can demonstrate both the presence of sites of increased metabolic activity and of morphologic abnormalities.[40] In a recent study by Radan and colleagues,[40] ^{62}FDG-PET/CT studies of newly diagnosed primary gastric lymphoma (24 low-grade mucosa-associated lymphoid tissue, and 38 aggressive NHL) were assessed and compared with 27 controls. Gastric CT abnormalities and extragastric sites were recorded. Gastric FDG uptake was found in 55 (89%) of 62 patients with primary gastric lymphoma (71% mucosa-associated lymphoid tissue versus 100% aggressive NHL; $P < .001$) and 63% controls. SUVmax in FDG-avid primary gastric lymphomas was 15.3 ± 11.7 (5.4 ± 2.9 for mucosa-associated lymphoid tissue, versus 19.7 ± 11.5 for aggressive NHL; $P < .001$) and 4.6 ± 1.4 in the controls. The authors concluded that FDG uptake can be differentiated, in particular in the aggressive NHL group, from physiologic tracer activity based on SUVmax. Extragastric foci seen on FDG-PET and structural CT abnormalities were additional useful parameters of FDG-PET/CT assessment of primary gastric lymphoma.

INTRAPAPILLARY MUCINOUS NEOPLASM OF THE PANCREAS

Within the whole group of cystic pancreatic tumors, preoperative imaging including MR cholangiopancreatography and endoscopic ultrasound usually allows for the differentiation of three main lesions: (1) serous adenoma, (2) mucinous tumor, and (3) intraductal papillary mucinous neoplasm (IPMN).[52,53] Although radiologic follow-up for serous adenoma and resection of mucinous neoplasms are the common management approaches for the first two tumors, IPMN still represents a diagnostic dilemma, because it can be histologically classified as adenoma, in situ carcinoma, or invasive carcinoma. Unfortunately, these lesions cannot be differentiated with sufficient accuracy by conventional imaging techniques.[52] As such, most investigators currently consider IPMNs, at the very least, premalignant.[54] Surgical resection is advocated in most instances especially for a main duct–type IPMN. The extent of surgical resection, however, may be dependent on the degree of malignancy. Less radical organ-preserving resections, such as duodenum-preserving pancreatic head resection and spleen-preserving distal pancreatectomy, may be performed for nonmalignant lesions.[55] Moreover, conservative management may be a viable option for benign or borderline lesions in high-risk patients with a shorter life-expectancy because observational studies suggest a time-lag of at least 5 years for the progression from benign to malignant IPMNs.[56] Preoperative determination of malignancy in IPMNs using the conventional imaging techniques, however, is almost impossible.

In the current medical literature, there are some reports addressing the successful role of FDG-PET in the evaluation of IPMNs.[52,53,57–60] The use of FDG-PET in the management of cystic lesions of the pancreas was first reported by Sperti and colleagues[57] They retrospectively evaluated 56 patients with cystic lesions of the pancreas comparing FDG-PET with CT scans using a SUV greater than 2.5 as positive for malignancy. FDG-PET had a sensitivity and specificity of 94% and 97%, respectively, compared with CT with a sensitivity and specificity of 65% and 87%, respectively. The same group subsequently performed a prospective study of 50 patients with very similar results.[58] Regarding their results for IPMN alone, FDG-PET correctly distinguished all IPMNs as benign (eight of eight) or malignant (one of one) in their initial study.[57] In their second study, FDG-PET correctly diagnosed eight of eight benign and eight of eight malignant IPMNs.[58] In a more recent study by Mansour and colleagues[60] including 68 patients with cystic lesions of the pancreas, FDG-PET correctly diagnosed three of three benign and one of two malignant IPMNs. In a very recent study by Baiocchi and colleagues,[52] the authors reviewed seven patients with IPMN that were studied both with FDG-PET and MR cholangiopancreatography. Focal increased glycolytic activity was documented in two patients with SUVs of 6.7 and 9, respectively, whereas absence of FDG uptake in the neoplasm area was recorded in the remaining five cases. The final diagnosis was benign IPMN in the five cases and malignant IPMN in two that showed increased FDG uptake. FDG-PET scan correctly predicted the presence or absence of malignancy in all patients, whereas MR cholangiopancreatography failed to detect malignancy in three cases.

SUMMARY

Despite the fact that GIST, gallbladder carcinoma, gastric lymphoma, and intrapapillary mucinous neoplasm of the pancreas are rare tumors of the gastrointestinal tract, they seem to possess the same oncogenic signaling that more common cancers show (their addiction to sugar). As a result, imaging with FDG-PET has made a big impact in these diseases, especially in GIST in the evaluation of response to new molecular-targeted drugs, such as imatinib mesylate and sunitinib malate. In that context, FDG-PET has been used as an in vivo pharmacodynamic assay, a biomarker of therapeutic response, an indicator of primary and secondary resistance, and a predictor of clinical outcome.

The lessons learned from these trials have led to several breakthroughs in the understanding of cancer that have reshaped cancer research and revolutionized patient care. New paradigms, such as therapies tailored to the genetic profile of a patient's tumor, are becoming a reality, and these new concepts are now being extended to all cancers.

ACKNOWLEDGMENTS

The authors thank Iryna Rastarhuyeva, MD, and Leonid Syrkin for their assistance with the figures; all the members of the nuclear medicine, radiology, and multidisciplinary teams for their expertise and dedication to our patients; and all the patients and their families who contributed so much of themselves for the benefit of all cancer patients.

REFERENCES

1. Esteves FP, Schuster DM, Halkar RK. Gastrointestinal tract malignancies and positron emission tomography: an overview. Semin Nucl Med 2006;36(2): 169–81.
2. Warburg O. The Metabolism of Tumours. Investigations from the Kaiser-Wilhelm Institute for Biology, Berlin-Dahlem. London: Constable & Co. Ltd.; 1930.

3. Bui T, Thompson CB. Cancer's sweet tooth [comment]. Cancer Cell 2006;9(6):419–20.

4. Mazur MT, Clark HB. Gastric stromal tumors: reappraisal of histogenesis. Am J Surg Pathol 1983;7(6):507–19.

5. Kindblom LG, Aldenborg F, Meis-Kindblom JM, et al. Gastrointestinal pacemaker cell tumor (GIPACT): gastrointestinal stromal tumors show phenotypic characteristics of the interstitial cells of Cajal. Am J Pathol 1998;152(5):1259–69.

6. Hirota S, Isozaki K, Nishida T, et al. Effects of loss-of-function and gain-of-function mutations of c-kit on the gastrointestinal tract. J Gastroenterol 2000;35(Suppl 12):75–9.

7. Bucher P, Villiger P, Egger JF, et al. Management of gastrointestinal stromal tumors: from diagnosis to treatment. Swiss Med Wkly 2004;134(11–12):145–53.

8. Miettinen M, Lasota J. Gastrointestinal stromal tumors: definition, clinical, histological, immunohistochemical, and molecular genetic features and differential diagnosis. Virchows Arch 2001;438(1):1–12.

9. Blanchard DK, Budde JM, Hatch GF, et al. Tumors of the small intestine. World J Surg 2000;24(4):421–9.

10. Lau S, Tam KF, Kam CK, et al. Imaging of gastrointestinal stromal tumour (GIST). Clin Radiol 2004;59(6):487–98.

11. Connolly EM, Gaffney E, Reynolds JV. Gastrointestinal stromal tumours. Br J Surg 2003;90(10):1178–86.

12. DeMatteo RP. The GIST of targeted cancer therapy: a tumor (gastrointestinal stromal tumor), a mutated gene (c-kit), and a molecular inhibitor (STI571). Ann Surg Oncol 2002;9(9):831–9.

13. Fletcher CD, Berman JJ, Corless C, et al. Diagnosis of gastrointestinal stromal tumors: a consensus approach [see comment]. Hum Pathol 2002;33(5):459–65.

14. Lux ML, Rubin BP, Biase TL, et al. KIT extracellular and kinase domain mutations in gastrointestinal stromal tumors. Am J Pathol 2000;156(3):791–5.

15. Corless CL, Fletcher JA, Heinrich MC. Biology of gastrointestinal stromal tumors. J Clin Oncol 2004;22(18):3813–25.

16. Heinrich MC, Corless CL, Demetri GD, et al. Kinase mutations and imatinib response in patients with metastatic gastrointestinal stromal tumor. J Clin Oncol 2003;21(23):4342–9.

17. Heinrich MC, Corless CL, Duensing A, et al. PDGFRA activating mutations in gastrointestinal stromal tumors. Science 2003;299(5607):708–10.

18. Hirota S, Ohashi A, Nishida T, et al. Gain-of-function mutations of platelet-derived growth factor receptor alpha gene in gastrointestinal stromal tumors. Gastroenterology 2003;125(3):660–7.

19. Heinrich MC, Corless CL, Blanke CD, et al. Molecular correlates of imatinib resistance in gastrointestinal stromal tumors. J Clin Oncol 2006;24(29):4764–74.

20. Demetri GD, van Oosterom AT, Garrett CR, et al. Efficacy and safety of sunitinib in patients with advanced gastrointestinal stromal tumour after failure of imatinib: a randomised controlled trial. Lancet 2006;368(9544):1329–38.

21. Van den Abbeele AD, for the GIST Collaborative PET Study Group (Dana-Farber Cancer Institute, Boston, Massachusetts; OHSU, Portland, Oregon, Helsinki University Central Hospital, Turku University Central Hospital, Finland, Novartis Oncology). F18-FDG-PET provides early evidence of biological response to ST15171 in patients with malignant gastrointestinal stromal tumors (GIST). Proc Am Soc Clin Oncol 2001;20:362a.

22. Demetri GD, von Mehren M, Blanke CD, et al. Efficacy and safety of imatinib mesylate in advanced gastrointestinal stromal tumors. N Engl J Med 2002;347(7):472–80.

23. Van den Abbeele AD, Badawi RD. Use of positron emission tomography in oncology and its potential role to assess response to imatinib mesylate therapy in gastrointestinal stromal tumors (GISTs). Eur J Cancer 2002;38(Suppl 5):S60–5.

24. Dagher R, Cohen M, Williams G, et al. Approval summary: imatinib mesylate in the treatment of metastatic and/or unresectable malignant gastrointestinal stromal tumors. Clin Cancer Res 2002;8(10):3034–8.

25. Young H, Baum R, Cremerius U, et al. Measurement of clinical and subclinical tumour response using [18F]-fluorodeoxyglucose and positron emission tomography: review and 1999 EORTC recommendations. European Organization for Research and Treatment of Cancer (EORTC) PET study group. Eur J Cancer 1999;35(13):1773–82.

26. Holdsworth CH, Manola J, Badawi RD, et al. Use of computerized tomography (CT) as an early prognostic indicator of response to imatinib mesylate (IM) in patients with gastrointestinal stromal tumors (GIST). J Clin Oncol, 2004 ASCO Annual Meeting Proceedings (Post-Meeting Edition). Vol 22, No 14S (July 15 Supplement), 2004: 3011, 2004. 22(14S (July 15 Supplement)): p. 3011.

27. Stroobants S, Seegers M, Goeminne J, et al. 18FDG-positron emission tomography for the early prediction of response in advanced soft tissue sarcoma treated with imatinib mesylate (Glivec). Eur J Cancer 2003;39:2012–20.

28. Choi H, Charnsangavej C, Faria SC, et al. Correlation of computed tomography and positron emission tomography in patients with metastatic gastrointestinal stromal tumor treated at a single institution with imatinib mesylate: proposal of new computed

tomography response criteria. J Clin Oncol 2007; 25(13):1753–9.

29. Heinicke T, Wardelmann E, Sauerbruch T, et al. Very early detection of response to imatinib mesylate therapy of gastrointestinal stromal tumours using 18fluoro-deoxyglucose-positron emission tomography. Anticancer Res 2005;25(6C):4591–4.

30. Jager PL, Gietema JA, van der Graaf WT. Imatinib mesylate fro the treatment of gastrointestinal stromal tumours: best monitored with FDG PET. Nucl Med Commun 2004;25(5):433–8.

31. Goerres GW, Stupp R, Barghouth G, et al. The value of PET, CT and in-line PET/CT in patients with gastrointestinal stromal tumours: long-term outcome of treatment with imatinib mesylate. Eur J Nucl Med Mol Imaging 2005;32(2):153–62.

32. Antoch G, Kanja J, Bauer S, et al. Comparison of PET, CT, and dual-modality PET/CT imaging for monitoring of imatinib (ST1571) therapy in patients with gastrointestinal stromal tumors. J Nucl Med 2004;45(3):357–65.

33. Holdsworth CH, Badawi RD, Manola JB, et al. CT and PET: early prognostic indicators of response to imatinib mesylate in patients with gastrointestinal stromal tumor. AJR Am J Roentgenol 2007;189(6): W324–30.

34. Van den Abbeele AD, Badawi R, Manola J, et al. Effects of cessation of imatinib mesylate (IM) therapy in patients (pts) with IM-refractory gastrointestinal stromal tumors (GIST) as visualized by FDG-PET scanning. Proc Am Soc Clin Oncol 2004;22:3012.

35. Hirooka Y, Naitoh Y, Goto H, et al. Differential diagnosis of gall-bladder masses using colour Doppler ultrasonography. J Gastroenterol Hepatol 1996; 11(9):840–6.

36. Oe A, Kawabe J, Torii K, et al. Distinguishing benign from malignant gallbladder wall thickening using FDG-PET. Ann Nucl Med 2006;20(10):699–703.

37. Shukla HS. Gallbladder cancer. J Surg Oncol 2006; 93(8):604–6.

38. Rodriguez-Fernandez A, Gomez-Rio M, Llamas-Elvira JM, et al. Positron-emission tomography with fluorine-18-fluoro-2-deoxy-D-glucose for gallbladder cancer diagnosis. Am J Surg 2004;188(2):171–5.

39. Anderson CD, Rice MH, Pinson CW, et al. Fluorodeoxyglucose PET imaging in the evaluation of gallbladder carcinoma and cholangiocarcinoma. J Gastrointest Surg 2004;8(1):90–7.

40. Radan L, Fischer D, Bar-Shalom R, et al. FDG avidity and PET/CT patterns in primary gastric lymphoma. Eur J Nucl Med Mol Imaging 2008;35(8):1424–30.

41. d'Amore F, Brincker H, Gronbaek K, et al. Non-Hodgkin's lymphoma of the gastrointestinal tract: a population-based analysis of incidence, geographic distribution, clinicopathologic presentation features, and prognosis. Danish lymphoma study group. J Clin Oncol 1994;12(8):1673–84.

42. Akwaa A, Siddiqui N, Al-Mofleh I. Primary gastric lymphoma. World J Gastroenterol 2004;10:5–11.

43. Zucca E, Conconi A, Cavalli F. Treatment of extranodal lymphomas. Best Pract Res Clin Haematol 2002; 15(3):533–47.

44. Ambrosini V, Rubello D, Castellucci P, et al. Diagnostic role of 18F-FDG PET in gastric MALT lymphoma. Nucl Med Rev Cent East Eur 2006;9(1):37–40.

45. Kumar R, Xiu Y, Potenta S, et al. 18F-FDG PET for evaluation of the treatment response in patients with gastrointestinal tract lymphomas. J Nucl Med 2004;45(11):1796–803.

46. Phongkitkarun S, Varavithya V, Kazama T, et al. Lymphomatous involvement of gastrointestinal tract: evaluation by positron emission tomography with (18)F-fluorodeoxyglucose. World J Gastroenterol 2005;11(46):7284–9.

47. Beal KP, Yeung HW, Yahalom J. FDG-PET scanning for detection and staging of extranodal marginal zone lymphomas of the MALT type: a report of 42 cases. Ann Oncol 2005;16(3):473–80.

48. Schoder H, Noy A, Gonen M, et al. Intensity of 18fluorodeoxyglucose uptake in positron emission tomography distinguishes between indolent and aggressive non-Hodgkin's lymphoma. J Clin Oncol 2005;23(21):4643–51.

49. Hoffmann M, Kletter K, Becherer A, et al. 18F-fluorodeoxyglucose positron emission tomography (18F-FDG-PET) for staging and follow-up of marginal zone B-cell lymphoma. Oncology 2003;64(4): 336–40.

50. Even-Sapir E, Lievshitz G, Perry C, et al. Fluorine-18 fluorodeoxyglucose PET/CT patterns of extranodal involvement in patients with non-Hodgkin's lymphoma and Hodgkin's disease. PET Clin N Am 2006;1:251–63.

51. Metser U, Goor O, Lerman H, et al. PET-CT of extranodal lymphoma. AJR Am J Roentgenol 2004; 182(6):1579–86.

52. Baiocchi GL, Portolani N, Bertagna F, et al. Possible additional value of 18FDG-PET in managing pancreas intraductal papillary mucinous neoplasms: preliminary results. J Exp Clin Cancer Res 2008; 27:10.

53. Fernandez-del Castillo C, Warshaw AL. Cystic tumors of the pancreas. Surg Clin North Am 1995; 75(5):1001–16.

54. Goh BK, Chung YF, Ng DC, et al. Positron emission tomography with 2-deoxy-2-[18f] fluoro-D-glucose in the detection of malignancy in intraductal papillary mucinous neoplasms of the pancreas. JOP 2007; 8(3):350–4.

55. Jang JY, Kim SW, Ahn YJ, et al. Multicenter analysis of clinicopathologic features of intraductal papillary mucinous tumor of the pancreas: is it possible to predict the malignancy before surgery? Ann Surg Oncol 2005;12(2):124–32.

56. Goh BK, Tan YM, Cheow PC, et al. Cystic lesions of the pancreas: an appraisal of an aggressive resectional policy adopted at a single institution during 15 years. Am J Surg 2006;192(2):148–54.

57. Sperti C, Pasquali C, Chierichetti F, et al. Value of 18-fluorodeoxyglucose positron emission tomography in the management of patients with cystic tumors of the pancreas. Ann Surg 2001;234(5):675–80.

58. Sperti C, Pasquali C, Decet G, et al. F-18-fluoro-deoxyglucose positron emission tomography in differentiating malignant from benign pancreatic cysts: a prospective study. J Gastrointest Surg 2005;9(1):22–8 [discussion 28–9].

59. Yoshioka M, Sato T, Furuya T, et al. Positron emission tomography with 2-deoxy-2-[(18)F] fluoro-d-glucose for diagnosis of intraductal papillary mucinous tumor of the pancreas with parenchymal invasion. J Gastroenterol 2003;38(12):1189–93.

60. Mansour JC, Schwartz L, Pandit-Taskar N, et al. The utility of F-18 fluorodeoxyglucose whole body PET imaging for determining malignancy in cystic lesions of the pancreas. J Gastrointest Surg 2006;10(10):1354–60.

Therapy Monitoring with Fluorine-18 FDG-PET and Fluorine-18 FDG-PET/CT

Hinrich A. Wieder, MD[a],*, Ken Herrmann, MD[b]

KEYWORDS

- FDG • PET-CT • Gastrointestinal cancer
- Therapy monitoring

Changes in tumor size have been used to assess tumor response in patients with gastrointestinal cancer. According to criteria of the World Health Organization (WHO), tumors should be measured in two perpendicular diameters. Tumor response is defined as a therapy-induced reduction of the product of these two diameters by at least 50%. In 2000, Therasse and colleagues[1] published newer guidelines called Response Evaluation Criteria for Solid Tumors (RECIST). RECIST characterized target lesions and nontarget lesions, which are used to extrapolate an overall response to treatment. In addition, the bidimensional measurements required by the WHO criteria have been replaced by unidimensional measurements. RECIST defines response as a 30% decrease of the largest diameter of the tumor. For a spherical lesion, this is equivalent to a 50% decrease of the product of two diameters. Meta-analyses combining the results of several large phase II and phase III studies have shown that tumor response according to WHO or RECIST criteria correlates with patient survival for some tumor types.[2] However, there is a considerable variability between individual studies and the same response rate can be associated with completely different survival rates in different studies.[3] For some tumor types, meta-analyses found no or only very weak correlation with patient survival.[4,5]

In addition to size measurements, tumor response has also been evaluated histopathologically. A common criterion for histopathological response to therapy is the absence of tumor cells or the presence of only scattered tumor cells (<10% viable tumor cells) in the resected specimen.[6] In a neoadjuvant (preoperative) setting, the overall survival of patients strongly depends on whether or not histopathological response is achieved. However, because of the tumor heterogeneity after neoadjuvant therapy, small biopsies of the tumor tissue are not representative of the whole tumor mass. A complete tumor resection and a histopathological examination of the whole tumor, including adjoining areas, is needed to definitely determine the histopathological tumor response. Thus, histopathological response can only be determined for patients undergoing preoperative chemo- or radiotherapy and it cannot be used to modify treatment.

The reproducibility of the positron emission tomography (PET) signal arising from fluorine-18 fluorodeoxyglucose ([18F]-FDG) accumulation in tumors has been shown to be rather stable at repeated examinations.[7] The interstudy variability

[a] Department of Radiology, Klinikum rechts der Isar, Technische Universität München, 22, 81675 München, Germany
[b] Department of Nuclear Medicine, Klinikum rechts der Isar, Technische Universität München, 22, 81675 München, Germany
* Corresponding author.
E-mail address: h@wieder.de (H.A. Wieder).

PET Clin 3 (2008) 217–226
doi:10.1016/j.cpet.2008.08.009

of repeated [18F]-FDG measurements within 3 weeks is less than 20%. In other words, during therapy, any change in tumor [18F]-FDG uptake greater than 20% between baseline PET and follow-up PET must be considered a true one. For example, a decrease of more than 20% can be seen as a therapeutic effect.

A high number of clinical studies have recently evaluated the role of [18F]-FDG PET for assessment of therapy response and tumor control and for prediction of prognosis. Imaging with [18F]-FDG PET appears to be especially promising as a clinical tool for evaluating response to therapy.

Studies evaluating treatment monitoring with [18F]-FDG PET can be divided into two groups.[8]

In the first, tumor response was assessed by [18F]-FDG PET after completion of chemo- or radiotherapy. Imaging with [18F]-FDG PET was performed several months after start of therapy and residual tumor [18F]-FDG uptake or changes in [18F]-FDG uptake from a pretherapeutic scan were correlated with histopathologic response or patient survival or both.

In the second group of studies [18F]-FDG PET scans were acquired before therapy and repeated during or immediately after the first chemotherapy cycle (2–4 weeks after start of therapy). Changes in [18F]-FDG uptake from the pretherapeutic scan to the early follow-up scan were then used to predict subsequent reduction of tumor size, histopathologic response, or patient survival. Data analyses are generally different between these two groups of studies. After completion of chemo- or radiotherapy, [18F]-FDG uptake of responding tumors should have decreased to background levels and focal [18F]-FDG uptake generally indicates macroscopic viable tumor tissue. Quantitative analysis is frequently not required at this time. However, quantitative assessment of tumor metabolism becomes necessary when [18F]-FDG PET scans are performed during treatment to predict subsequent tumor response. At this time, the metabolic activity of the tumor tissue has decreased in responders, but generally there will be still considerable residual [18F]-FDG uptake.

The following section gives an overview of the role of [18F]-FDG PET and [18F]-FDG PET/CT in the assessment of therapy response and prognosis with special emphasis on the early therapy response evaluation in patients with gastrointestinal cancer.

ESOPHAGEAL CANCER

In 2001, Brucher and colleagues[9] were the first to report a study evaluating [18F]-FDG PET for the assessment of a late metabolic response after completion of chemoradiotherapy in 27 patients with advanced squamous cell carcinoma of the esophagus. The patients underwent an [18F]-FDG PET scan before therapy and 3 to 4 weeks after completion of therapy. Therapy-induced reduction of tumor [18F]-FDG uptake was significantly higher for histopathologic responders (72% ± 11%) than for nonresponders (42% ± 22%). At a threshold of 52% decrease of metabolic activity, sensitivity to detect histopathologic response was 100%, with a corresponding specificity of 55%. Metabolic tumor response was also a strong prognostic parameter. Responders to [18F]-FDG PET scanning had a median survival of 23 months, whereas median survival was only 9 months in [18F]-FDG PET nonresponders. Similar results were obtained by Flamen and colleagues.[10] They studied 36 patients with esophageal cancer before and 3 to 4 weeks after completion of chemoradiotherapy. In contrast to the study by Brucher and colleagues, Flamen and colleagues' assessments of [18F]-FDG PET response were based on visual analysis. Patients were classified as [18F]-FDG PET responders if they showed a complete or almost complete normalization of the [18F]-FDG uptake at the primary site of the tumor together with a complete normalization of all lymph node metastases seen on the first [18F]-FDG PET scan before therapy. Histopathologic response was detected with a sensitivity of 78% and a specificity of 82% by [18F]-FDG PET. However, the sensitivity and the positive predictive value of the [18F]-FDG PET scan for the diagnosis of a complete histopathologic response were only 67% and 50%, respectively. The investigators stated that the underestimation of complete histopathological response by [18F]-FDG PET was mainly based on false-positive findings at the primary tumor site. An influx of leucocytes and macrophages due to inflammatory immune and scavenging reactions may increase the [18F]-FDG uptake, resulting in an underestimation of therapeutic efficacy. Again, metabolic response was also correlated with overall survival. The median overall survival for patients without an [18F]-FDG PET response was 6.4 months, whereas it was 16.4 months for patients classified as [18F]-FDG PET responders. Port and colleagues[11] compared in 62 patients with esophageal carcinoma [18F]-FDG PET response to clinical response for prediction of pathologic downstaging and disease-free survival. A reduction of primary tumor standardized uptake values (SUV_{max}) of more than 50% compared with baseline was more significantly associated with improved disease-free survival than clinical response. Regarding prediction of pathologic downstaging, the methods appeared to be equally accurate. However, Port and colleagues[11] showed that a complete absence of residual [18F]-FDG uptake cannot be equated with a complete pathologic response. This observation confirmed an earlier published study by Swisher and colleagues[12] involving 103 patients. This study proved that [18F]-FDG PET failed to rule out residual microscopic disease by showing that [18F]-FDG uptake in the tumor bed was the same for patients with no residual viable tumor cells as for patients with up to 10% viable tumor cells. Swisher and colleagues also investigated prognostic relevance of [18F]-FDG uptake after completion of neoadjuvant chemoradiation, claiming that a residual uptake of greater than SUV 4 was the best long-term survival predictor (hazard ratio 3.5, $P = .04$). Accuracy of [18F]-FDG PET for prediction of histopathological response was comparable to CT and ultrasound. In contrast to these results, Smithers and colleagues[13] found in 45 patients undergoing neoadjuvant chemotherapy or chemoradiation no correlation between [18F]-FDG PET response and histopathological response. These conflicting reported results underline the need for randomized multicenter studies with standardized imaging protocols, such as the studies recently launched by the European Organization for Research on Treatment of Cancer.[14]

Future approaches will try to combine metabolic information determined by [18F]-FDG PET with biological markers. Westerterp and colleagues[15] assessed in 26 patients [18F]-FDG uptake as well as stained biopsy tissue samples immunhistochemical for angiogenic markers (vascular endothelial cell growth factor, CD31), glucose transporter-1, hexokinase isoforms, proliferation marker (Ki67), macrophage marker (CD68), and apoptosis marker (cleaved caspase-3). The only parameters associated with [18F]-FDG uptake were glucose transporter-1 expression and tumor size.

Using quantitative measurements of tumor [18F]-FDG uptake, it is feasible not only to assess tumor response late after onset of therapy but also to predict response early during chemotherapy. In a study by Weber and colleagues,[16] 40 consecutive patients with an adenocarcinomas of the esophagogastric junction (AEG) had an [18F]-FDG PET scan before chemotherapy and on day 14 of the first chemotherapy cycle. The reduction of tumor [18F]-FDG uptake after 14 days of therapy was significantly different between tumors that showed a clinical and histopathological response and those that showed no response. Optimal differentiation was achieved by a cutoff value of 35% reduction of initial [18F]-FDG uptake. Applying this cut-off value as a criterion for a metabolic

response predicted clinical response with a sensitivity and specificity of 93% and 95%, respectively. Histopathologically complete or subtotal tumor regression was observed in 53% of the patients with a metabolic response but only in 5% of the patients without a metabolic response. Patients with a metabolic response were also characterized by a significantly longer time to progression/recurrence and longer overall survival (**Fig. 1** and **2**).

However, there is currently no consensus on the most appropriate time for monitoring tumor response by [18F]-FDG PET. To address this question, Wieder and colleagues[17] studied 24 patients with [18F]-FDG PET before chemotherapy (PET1), 2 weeks after start of chemotherapy (PET2), and 3 to 4 weeks after completion of chemotherapy (PET3). The relative decrease of tumor [18F]-FDG uptake from PET1 to PET2 and from PET1 to PET3 significantly correlated with histopathologic response for both time points. Reduction of tumor SUV from PET1 to PET2 significantly correlated with survival ($P = .03$) and there was a similar trend for changes from PET1 to PET3 ($P = .09$). Therefore, metabolic changes within the first 2 weeks of therapy are at least as efficient for prediction of histopathologic response and patient survival as later changes.

Based on the findings by Weber and colleagues,[16] treatment was tailored to the individual patient in dependence of the PET results in the recently published MUNICON trial.[18] This prospective, single-center study recruited 119 patients with locally advanced adenocarcinoma of AEG type 1 (distal esophageal adenocarcinoma) or type 2 (gastric cardia adenocarcinoma). All patients were assigned to 2 weeks of platinum- and fluorouracil-based induction chemotherapy (evaluation period). Metabolic responders after 2 weeks of induction chemotherapy continued to receive chemotherapy for a maximum of 12 weeks before undergoing surgery, whereas metabolic nonresponders discontinued chemotherapy and were immediately transferred to surgery after only 2 weeks of chemotherapy. In this trial, 110 patients were evaluable for metabolic response and 49% were classified as metabolic responders after 2 weeks of induction chemotherapy; 104 patients had tumor resection. Histopathological response was achieved in 58% of the metabolic responders, but in none of the metabolic nonresponders. After a median follow-up of 2.3 years, survival analysis revealed better event-free and overall survival for metabolic responders than for nonresponders (29.7 event-free months for metabolic responders versus 14.1 event-free months for nonresponders, $P = .002$; and overall survival not reached for metabolic

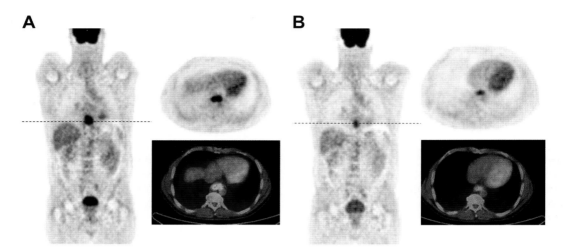

Fig. 1. Coronal PET (*A and B, left*), axial PET (*A and B, top right*), and PET-CT fusion (*A and B, bottom right*) images of a patient with locally advanced AEG. Already 14 days after initiation of neoadjuvant chemotherapy, there is a marked decrease in tumor metabolic activity (>35%). After completion of chemotherapy, no viable tumor cells were found in the resected specimen.

responders versus overall survival of 25.8 months for nonresponders, $P = .015$). This study confirmed prospectively the usefulness of early metabolic response evaluation, and shows the feasibility of an [18F]-FDG PET–guided treatment algorithm. The findings might enable tailoring of multimodal treatment in accordance with individual tumor biology in future randomized trials.

Radiotherapy and chemoradiotherapy often cause local inflammatory reactions in the esophagus. Uptake of [18F]-FDG in inflammatory lesions is a commonly known phenomenon. Uptake of [18F]-FDG due to radiation-induced inflammation may limit the use of [18F]-FDG PET for metabolic monitoring of esophageal carcinomas as observed in late-response assessment with [18F]-FDG PET (see above). Therefore, it has been recommended that [18F]-FDG PET should be further postponed and only be performed several weeks or even months after completion of radiotherapy to assess tumor response. However, these recommendations are not based on systematic clinical data, but only on theoretic considerations and a few case reports. Wieder and colleagues[19] studied

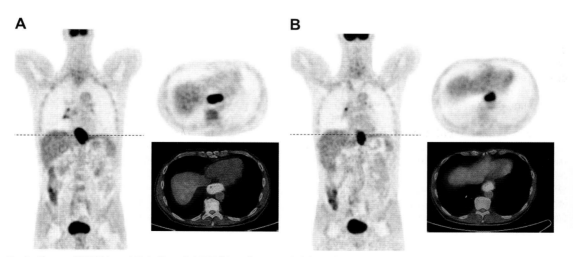

Fig. 2. Coronal PET (*A and B, left*), axial PET (*A and B, top right*), and PET-CT fusion (*A and B, bottom right*) images of a patient with locally advanced AEG. Fourteen days after initiation of neoadjuvant chemotherapy, there is a marginal decrease in tumor metabolic activity (<35%). After completion of chemotherapy, more than 50% of tumor cells were found in the resected specimen.

the time course of changes in tumor [18F]-FDG uptake in 38 patients with locally advanced squamous cell carcinomas of the esophagus during preoperative chemoradiotherapy. Patients underwent [18F]-FDG PET scans before chemoradiotherapy, 2 weeks after the initiation of therapy, and 3 to 4 weeks after completion of chemoradiotherapy (ie, before surgery). None of the serial [18F]-FDG PET scans demonstrated a relevant increase in tumor [18F]-FDG uptake, indicating that, because of therapy-induced loss of viable tumor cells, radiation-induced inflammation is too small to outweigh the decrease in [18F]-FDG uptake. Furthermore, radiation-induced esophagitis often involves a long segment of the esophagus and, in most cases, is markedly different from the [18F]-FDG uptake in esophageal cancer. Therefore, it is mostly possible to differentiate between residual tumor tissue and radiation-induced inflammation. The reduction of tumor [18F]-FDG uptake after 14 days of chemoradiotherapy was significantly higher in histopathologic responding tumors (44% ± 15%) than in nonresponders (21% ± 14%). The receiver operating curve analysis demonstrated that the highest accuracy for differentiation of subsequently responding and nonresponding tumors was achieved by applying a cutoff of a 30% decrease in tumor [18F]-FDG uptake from baseline values. Applying this cutoff value as a criterion for metabolic response allowed for prediction of histopathologic response with a sensitivity and a specificity of 93% and 88%, respectively. Patients with a metabolic response were also characterized by a significantly longer overall survival. The median overall survival for patients with a decrease in [18F] FDG uptake by more than 30% was more than 38 months, while it was 18 months for patients with a decrease of less than 30%. Thus, response prediction is clearly feasible with [18F]-FDG PET early in the course of chemoradiotherapy.

This is the basis for individualizing therapy (ie, continuing therapy in patients with tumor response and intensifying or aborting ineffective therapy in cases without response).

In a more recent publication by Gillham and colleagues,[20] response evaluation was assessed already 1 week after start of chemoradiation. However, [18F]-FDG PET failed to predict histomorphological tumor response in this study cohort of 32 patients (5 squamous cell carcinoma, 27 AEG).

GASTRIC CANCER

As nicely summarized by Ott and colleagues[21] in a recently published review, current imaging

modalities or molecular markers cannot reliably predict therapy response before or early in the course of treatment of patients with gastric cancer. Early assessment of response to neoadjuvant chemotherapy was first studied by Ott and colleagues[22] in 44 patients with locally advanced gastric cancer. Using the same criterion for differentiating metabolic responders and nonresponders as defined by Weber and colleagues[16] for patients with AEG, early response assessment by [18F]-FDG PET turned out to predict histopathological response with a sensitivity of 77% and specificity of 86% respectively. Median survival and 2-year survival rate were significantly better for metabolic responders (not reached and 90%) than for nonresponders (18.9 months and 25%; $P = .002$). In this study, approximately one third of gastric cancer patients had initially an [18F]-FDG uptake insufficient for quantification. Further analysis showed that [18F]-FDG–nonavid tumors are associated with diffuse Lauren classification, small tumor size, good differentiation, mucinous content, and localization in the distal third. Recently published long-term results claim that in locally advanced gastric cancer, three different metabolic groups exist.[23] Metabolic responders had a higher histopathological response rate (69%) than metabolic nonresponders (17%) and initially non–[18F]-FDG–avid patients (24%). Survival of non–[18F]-FDG–avid patients was not significantly different from that of [18F]-FDG–avid nonresponders (36.7 months versus 24.1 months; $P = .46$), whereas for [18F]-FDG–avid responders, median overall survival was not reached yet. Ott and colleagues[23] therefore assume that even though metabolic response assessment is not possible in non–[18F]-FDG–avid tumors, a therapy modification might be considered in this patient subgroup. Another group investigated a different time point and cutoff value in 41 patients with gastric cancer.[24] In this retrospective study, a decrease of more than 45% of the initial SUV after 35 days was revealed to be the best criterion for predicting response and prognosis to preoperative chemotherapy. Metabolic response was significantly correlated with histopathological response (less than 50% residual tumor; $P = .007$) and disease-free survival ($P = .01$). Again, a routine use of these parameters in a clinical setting cannot be established before a standardization of this methodology and prospective evaluation in a multicenter trial has been effected. Because around a third of gastric carcinomas are [18F]-FDG nonavid and therefore not suitable for response monitoring using [18F]-FDG PET, [18F]-fluorothymidine ([18F]-FLT) PET has been studied for detection of locally advanced gastric cancer by our group.[25]

Even though absolute uptake values were lower for [18F]-FLT than for [18F]-FDG, [18F]-FLT PET revealed a higher sensitivity than that for [18F]-FDG PET and might serve as a useful diagnostic adjunct reflecting the quantitative assessment of proliferation. In the future, the addition of [18F]-FLT PET to [18F]-FDG PET could improve the early evaluation of response to neoadjuvant treatment of gastric cancer.

COLORECTAL CANCER

Therapy response was first evaluated by Findlay and colleagues[26] in liver metastases of colorectal cancer showing that changes of [18F]-FDG uptake were correlated with the antitumor effect in chemotherapy. Early response assessment after initiation of chemoradiotherapy was studied by Cascini and colleagues[27] in 33 patients with locally advanced rectal cancer. Patients underwent [18F]-FDG PET scans before start of therapy and 12 days after starting treatment. Half of the included patients had a third [18F]-FDG PET scan before surgery. Retrospective receiver operating curve analysis revealed that a cutoff of 52% mean SUV decrease separated histologic responders from nonresponders with a high sensitivity, specificity, and accuracy (100%, 87%, and 94% respectively). The use of [18F]-FDG PET after completion of chemoradiotherapy was also investigated in recently published studies. Calvo and colleagues[28] investigated the prognostic value of the SUV_{max} 4 to 5 weeks after completion of chemoradiotherapy in patients with locally advanced rectal cancer. Presurgical SUV_{max} below or above 2.5 did not discriminate for recurrence or patient outcome. In contrast, initial SUV_{max} of less than 6 was correlated with a significantly better 3-year overall survival than for the group with a SUV_{max} of 6 or more (93% versus 60%, $P = .04$). In a study by Guillem and colleagues,[29] 15 patients with locally advanced rectal cancer underwent an [18F]-FDG PET scan before and 4 to 5 weeks after completion of neoadjuvant chemoradiotherapy. A reduction of SUV mean of more than 62.5% was defined as metabolic response and correlated significantly with better recurrence-free survival ($P = .02$). In a more recent study, 44 patients with primary rectal cancer and 4 patients with pelvic recurrence underwent [18F]-FDG PET scans before start of neoadjuvant chemoradiotherapy and 5 to 6 weeks after completion.[30] Receiver operating curve analysis revealed a decrease of 66.5% SUV_{max} compared with baseline as optimal cutoff, resulting in a sensitivity of 81%, a specificity of 79% and an overall accuracy of 80%, respectively. The results of these studies suggest the potential utility of [18F]-FDG PET as

a complementary diagnostic and prognostic procedure in the assessment of neoadjuvant chemoradiotherapy response of locally advanced rectal cancer. An evaluation has also been made for [18F]-FDG PET in assessing response to palliative chemotherapy in 50 patients with metastatic colorectal cancer. These patients received [18F]-FDG PET scans initially and after 2 and 6 months into treatment.[31] The study showed that change of both, metabolic rate of glucose (cutoff: 65% decrease) and SUV (cutoff: 20% decrease) between the initial and the 2-month scan, were correlated with overall survival ($P = .009$ and $P = .021$, respectively).

Similar results were found in a more recent study by Rosenberg and colleagues[32] in 30 patients with locally advanced rectal cancer undergoing neoadjuvant chemoradiotherapy. Metabolic response evaluation by PET-CT was performed 2 weeks after start of chemoradiotherapy and after completion of chemoradiotherapy before surgery (**Fig. 3 and 4**). Receiver operating curve analysis resulted in optimal cutoffs of 35% and 57.5% SUV decrease for the early and late time point respectively, leading to a sensitivity of 74% and 79% respectively. Corresponding specificity was 70% for both time points. Rosenberg and colleagues attributed the reduced sensitivity to nonmalignant FDG uptake due to chemoradiotherapy-induced inflammation. Evaluation of early metabolic response assessment should be studied in larger patient groups possibly leading to modification or avoidance of ineffective treatment.

However, in rectal cancer, [18F]-FDG PET is limited by the high activity concentration in the bladder, which can cause artifacts. Furthermore, local inflammatory reactions are common after radiotherapy of rectal cancer. Increased [18F]-FDG uptake in inflammation may also limit the accuracy of [18F]-FDG PET in evaluating rectal cancer immediately following chemoradiotherapy. Wieder and colleagues[33] evaluated whether PET imaging with [11C]methyl-L-methionine (MET) may be used to monitor the response of rectal cancer to preoperative chemoradiotherapy. The potential advantages of MET over [18F]-FDG are the lower renal clearance that results in a lower tracer concentration in the bladder, which may facilitate detection of rectal cancer. It has also been previously shown that, in some animal models, inflamed tissues have a lower uptake of MET than of [18F]-FDG.[19] Therefore, after radiotherapy, the rate of false-positive findings with [11C]-MET PET may be lower than that with [18F]-FDG PET. Tumor response was assessed by the change in tumor (T) stage during therapy and by the percentage of viable tumor cells in the histopathological specimen

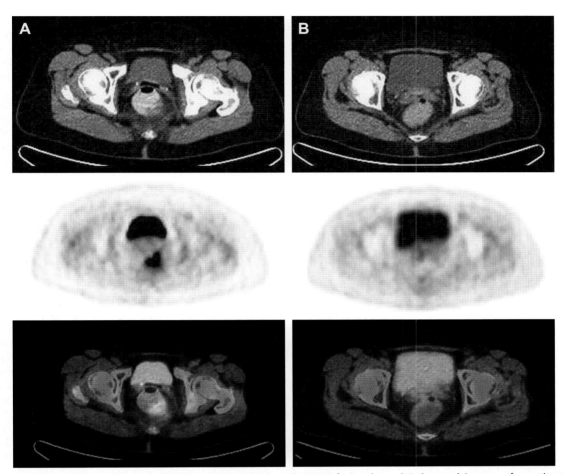

Fig. 3. Axial CT (*A* and *B, top*), PET (*A* and *B, middle*), and PET-CT fusion (*A* and *B, bottom*) images of a patient with locally advanced rectal cancer. Already 12 days after initiation of neoadjuvant chemoradiotherapy, there is a marked decrease in tumor metabolic activity (>35%). After completion of chemoradiotherapy, the tumor was classified as histopathological responder.

after therapy. For the evaluation of the changes in T stage, the preoperative T stage in MR imaging was compared with the postoperative histopathological T stage.

In 15 patients, [11C]-MET PET was performed before and after preoperative chemoradiotherapy. After completion of chemoradiotherapy, 7 of the 15 patients showed a decrease in T stage and 7 patients at least a subtotal tumor regression. When a change in T stage was used as a criterion for response, no significant differences were found between responding and nonresponding tumors with respect to SUV before therapy ($P = .91$) or SUV after completion of therapy ($P = .91$). Furthermore, the change in [11C]-MET uptake during therapy ($P = .73$) did not correlate with response. The decrease in the mean SUVs of the responders during therapy was 55%, whereas it was 52% among the nonresponders. Similar results were

observed when response was assessed by histopathological response.

Therefore, [11C]-MET PET did not allow an assessment of the response to therapy.

In another study by Wieder and colleagues,[34] chemoradiotherapy also caused a marked decrease in [18F]-FLT uptake in patients with rectal cancer in both responding and nonresponding tumors, indicating that [18F]-FLT PET does not allow assessment of tumor response.

GASTROINTESTINAL STROMAL TUMORS

Stroobants and colleagues[35] evaluated the role of [18F]-FDG PET for early response evaluation to treatment with imatinib in a group of 21 patients with soft tissue sarcoma. Response to [18F]-FDG PET, defined according to the European Organization for Research and Treatment of Cancer

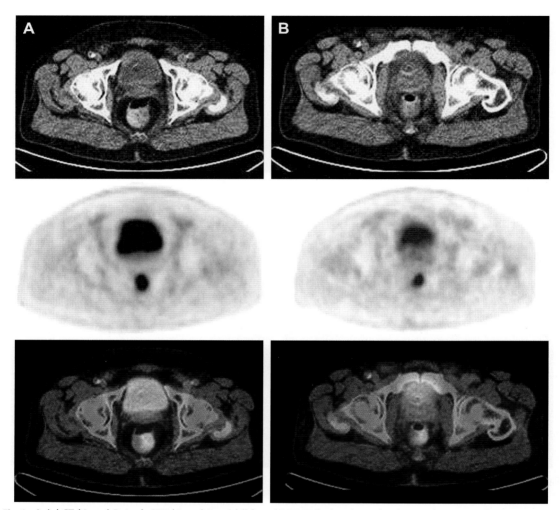

Fig. 4. Axial CT (*A and B, top*), PET (*A and B, middle*) and PET-CT fusion (*A and B, bottom*) images of a patient with locally advanced rectal cancer. Twelve days after initiation of neoadjuvant chemoradiotherapy, there is a marginal decrease in tumor metabolic activity (<35%). After completion of chemoradiotherapy, the tumor was classified as histopathological nonresponder.

[18F]-FDG PET recommendations, as early as at day 8 after initiation of imatinib treatment was associated with a significantly longer progression-free survival (1-year progression-free survival: 92% versus 12%, P = .001). Subsequent CT response (RECIST) was observed in 10 of these patients after a median follow-up of 8 weeks. Stable or progressive disease was observed on [18F]-FDG PET in 8 patients and none of them achieved a response on CT. Response evaluation by [18F]-FDG PET preceded CT response by a median of 7 weeks (range: 4–48).

REFERENCES

1. Therasse P, Arbuck SG, Eisenhauer EA, et al. New guidelines to evaluate the response to treatment in solid tumors. European Organization for Research and Treatment of Cancer, National Cancer Institute of the United States, National Cancer Institute of Canada. J Natl Cancer Inst 2000;92(3):205–16.
2. Buyse M, Piedbois Y, Piedbois P, et al. Tumour site, sex, and survival in colorectal cancer. Lancet 2000; 356(9232):858.
3. Bruzzi P, Del ML, Sormani MP, et al. Objective response to chemotherapy as a potential surrogate end point of survival in metastatic breast cancer patients. J Clin Oncol 2005;23(22):5117–25.
4. Goffin J, Baral S, Tu D, et al. Objective responses in patients with malignant melanoma or renal cell cancer in early clinical studies do not predict regulatory approval. Clin Cancer Res 2005;11(16):5928–34.
5. Ratain MJ. Phase II oncology trials: let's be positive. Clin Cancer Res 2005;11(16):5661–2.

6. Becker K, Mueller JD, Schulmacher C, et al. Histomorphology and grading of regression in gastric carcinoma treated with neoadjuvant chemotherapy. Cancer 2003;98(7):1521–30.
7. Weber WA, Ziegler SI, Thodtmann R, et al. Reproducibility of metabolic measurements in malignant tumors using FDG PET. J Nucl Med 1999;40(11):1771–7.
8. Weber WA, Wieder H. Monitoring chemotherapy and radiotherapy of solid tumors. Eur J Nucl Med Mol Imaging 2006;(33 Suppl 1):27–37.
9. Brücher BL, Weber W, Bauer M, et al. Neoadjuvant therapy of esophageal squamous cell carcinoma: response evaluation by positron emission tomography. Ann Surg 2001;233(3):300–9.
10. Flamen P, Van Cutsem E, Lerut A, et al. Positron emission tomography for assessment of the response to induction radiochemotherapy in locally advanced oesophageal cancer. Ann Oncol 2002;13(3):361–8.
11. Port JL, Lee PC, Korst RJ, et al. Positron emission tomographic scanning predicts survival after induction chemotherapy for esophageal carcinoma. Ann Thorac Surg 2007;84(2):393–400.
12. Swisher SG, Maish M, Erasmus JJ, et al. Utility of PET, CT, and EUS to identify pathologic responders in esophageal cancer. Ann Thorac Surg 2004;78(4):1152–60.
13. Smithers BM, Couper GC, Thomas JM, et al. Positron emission tomography and pathological evidence of response to neoadjuvant therapy in adenocarcinoma of the esophagus. Dis Esophagus 2008;21(2):151–8.
14. Lordick F, Ruers E, Aust DE, et al. European Organisation of Research and Treatment of Cancer (EORTC) Gastrointestinal Group: Workshop on the role of metabolic imaging in the neoadjuvant treatment of gastrointestinal cancer. Eur J Cancer 2008;13(44):1807–19.
15. Westerterp M, Sloof GW, Hoekstra OS, et al. 18FDG uptake in oesophageal adenocarcinoma: linking biology and outcome. J Cancer Res Clin Oncol 2008;134(2):227–36.
16. Weber WA, Ott K, Becker K, et al. Prediction of response to preoperative chemotherapy in adenocarcinomas of the esophagogastric junction by metabolic imaging. J Clin Oncol 2001;19(12):3058–65.
17. Wieder HA, Ott K, Lordick F, et al. Prediction of tumor response by FDG-PET: comparison of the accuracy of single and sequential studies in patients with adenocarcinomas of the esophagogastric junction. Eur J Nucl Med Mol Imaging 2007;34(12):1925–32.
18. Lordick F, Ott K, Krause BJ, et al. PET to assess early metabolic response and to guide treatment of adenocarcinoma of the oesophagogastric junction: the MUNICON phase II trial. Lancet Oncol 2007;8(9):797–805.
19. Wieder HA, Brucher BL, Zimmermann F, et al. Time course of tumor metabolic activity during chemoradiotherapy of esophageal squamous cell carcinoma and response to treatment. J Clin Oncol 2004;22(5):900–8.
20. Gillham CM, Lucey JA, Keogan M, et al. (18)FDG uptake during induction chemoradiation for oesophageal cancer fails to predict histomorphological tumour response. Br J Cancer 2006;95(9):1174–9.
21. Ott K, Lordick F, Herrmann K, et al. The new credo: induction chemotherapy in locally advanced gastric cancer: consequences for surgical strategies. Gastric Cancer 2008;11(1):1–9.
22. Ott K, Fink U, Becker K, et al. Prediction of response to preoperative chemotherapy in gastric carcinoma by metabolic imaging: results of a prospective trial. J Clin Oncol 2003;21(24):4604–10.
23. Ott K, Herrmann K, Lordick F, et al. Early metabolic response evaluation by fluorine-18 fluorodeoxyglucose positron emission tomography allows in vivo testing of chemosensitivity in gastric cancer: long-term results of a prospective study. Clin Cancer Res 2008;14(7):2012–8.
24. Shah MA, Yeung HW, Coit D, et al. A phase II study of preoperative chemotherapy with irinotecan (CPT) and cisplatin (CIS) for gastric cancer (NCI 5917): FDG-PET/CT predicts patient outcome. J Clin Oncol 2007;25:4502 [Ref Type: Abstract].
25. Herrmann K, Ott K, Buck AK, et al. Imaging gastric cancer with PET and the radiotracers 18F-FLT and 18F-FDG: a comparative analysis. J Nucl Med 2007;48(12):1945–50.
26. Findlay M, Young H, Cunningham D, et al. Noninvasive monitoring of tumor metabolism using fluorodeoxyglucose and positron emission tomography in colorectal cancer liver metastases: correlation with tumor response to fluorouracil. J Clin Oncol 1996;14(3):700–8.
27. Cascini GL, Avallone A, Delrio P, et al. 18F-FDG PET is an early predictor of pathologic tumor response to preoperative radiochemotherapy in locally advanced rectal cancer. J Nucl Med 2006;47(8):1241–8.
28. Calvo FA, Domper M, Matute R, et al. 18F-FDG positron emission tomography staging and restaging in rectal cancer treated with preoperative chemoradiation. Int J Radiat Oncol Biol Phys 2004;58(2):528–35.
29. Guillem JG, Moore HG, Akhurst T, et al. Sequential preoperative fluorodeoxyglucose-positron emission tomography assessment of response to preoperative chemoradiation: a means for determining long-term outcomes of rectal cancer. J Am Coll Surg 2004;199(1):1–7.
30. Funaioli C, Pinto C, Di FF, et al. 18FDG-PET evaluation correlates better than CT with pathological response in a metastatic colon cancer patient

treated with bevacizumab-based therapy. Tumori 2007;93(6):611–5.

31. de Geus-Oei LF, van Laarhoven HW, Visser EP, et al. Chemotherapy response evaluation with FDG-PET in patients with colorectal cancer. Ann Oncol 2008; 19(2):348–52.

32. Rosenberg R, Herrmann K, Gertler R, et al. Early and late metabolic response prediction to preoperative radiochemotherapy in locally advanced rectal cancer. Int J Colorectal Dis 2008 [Abstract].

33. Wieder H, Ott K, Zimmermann F, et al. PET imaging with [11C]methyl-L-methionine for therapy monitoring in patients with rectal cancer. Eur J Nucl Med Mol Imaging 2002;29(6):789–96.

34. Wieder HA, Geinitz H, Rosenberg R, et al. PET imaging with [(18)F]3'-deoxy-3'-fluorothymidine for prediction of response to neoadjuvant treatment in patients with rectal cancer. Eur J Nucl Med Mol Imaging 2007;34(6):878–83.

35. Stroobants SG, D'Hoore I, Dooms C, et al. Additional value of whole-body fluorodeoxyglucose positron emission tomography in the detection of distant metastases of non–small-cell lung cancer. Clin Lung Cancer 2003;4(4):242–7.

PET and PET/CT in Pediatric Gastrointestinal Tract Oncology

Wichana Chamroonrat, MD[a], Mohamed Houseni, MD[a,b],
Geming Li, MD[a], Abass Alavi, MD[a], Hongming Zhuang, MD, PhD[a,*]

KEYWORDS

- Pediatric oncology • Childhood malignancy
- PET • Gastrointestinal lymphoma
- Hepatoblastoma • Hyperinsulinism

Childhood cancers represent about 1% of all new cancer cases[1] and are the second highest cause of death (12.8%) in children in the United States.[2] Pediatric malignancies differ from adult neoplasms in both distribution and prognosis. Lymphohematopoietic cancers are the most common during childhood, as approximately 40% of all cancers. Nervous system cancers account for approximately 30%, and embryonal tumors and sarcomas account for approximately 20% of childhood cancers.[2] Childhood gastrointestinal malignancies include extranodal lymphoma of gastrointestinal tract; hepatic tumors; pancreatic tumors; and other rare neoplasms, such as gastrointestinal adenocarcinoma, biliary cancers, and gastric cancers. Metastases to gastrointestinal tract, although rare, may occur from neuroblastoma, Wilms' tumor, osteogenic sarcoma, and desmoplastic small round cell tumor.[3–5] Unlike incidence patterns in adults, there is a relatively wide age range in the pediatric age group, with two peaks, the first in early childhood and the second in adolescence.[6] The 5-year disease-free survival and cure in most childhood cancer is about 80%. This high survival rate reflects progress in the understanding of tumor biology and incremental improvements in diagnosis and therapy.[7,8]

Imaging of tumor metabolism using positron emission tomography (PET) has been wildly successful.[9–16] Such functional imaging can be used together with anatomic imaging to diagnose, characterize, or monitor tumors before and after therapeutic treatment.[17,18] Furthermore, the introduction of combined PET with CT has been an advancement in diagnostic imaging allowing synergistic interpretation and precise anatomic localization of the metabolic information. In pediatric population, the scan time is critical and the use of CT for attenuation correction has shortened the scan time.[19] The role of PET imaging in pediatric malignancies is still evolving with limited literature.[19,20]

This article reviews PET imaging in pediatric gastrointestinal oncology with a special focus on gastrointestinal lymphoma, liver malignancies, and pancreatic tumors.

PATIENT PREPARATION

Undertaking examination on children can be challenging. Child preparation for PET imaging includes a sheet wrapped around the body, sand bags and holding devices for immobilization, reliable intravenous access, and bladder

---

The first two authors contributed equally to this article.

[a] Department of Radiology, The Children's Hospital of Philadelphia, 34th Street and Civic Center Boulevard, Philadelphia, PA 19104, USA

[b] Department of Radiology, National Liver Institute, Egypt

* Corresponding author.

E-mail address: zhuanghm@yahoo.com (H. Zhuang).

PET Clin 3 (2008) 227–238
doi:10.1016/j.cpet.2008.10.004
1556-8598/08/$ – see front matter © 2008 Elsevier Inc. All rights reserved.

pet.theclinics.com

catheterization to avoid discomfort and possible contamination.[21,22] Sedation may be used according to the guidelines of the Society of Nuclear Medicine, the American Academy of Pediatrics, and the American Society of Anesthesiology.[23,24] Sedation may potentially affect tracer biodistribution but it is not known to affect tumor metabolism. Parents may accompany their child.[25]

RADIATION DOSIMETRY

The recommended dose of fluorodeoxyglucose (FDG) for children ranges from 0.15 to 0.30 (5–10 MBq) mCi/kg with a total dose of 1 mCi (37 MBq) and not more than 20 mCi (750 MBq).[26] Ruotsalainen and colleagues[27] reported the absorbed radiation dose in a series of 21 infants. Bladder wall is the target organ. Absorbed dose per unit in variable organs of infants is higher than that reported in adults. The total body absorbed dose is lower in infants, however, compared with adults.[25,27] Using PET-CT, the radiation doses of the CT part using 80 mA and 140 kV is 3 to 5 mSv. The effective doses from diagnostic CT procedures are estimated to be of 1 to 10 mSv. The dose from a diagnostic CT procedure may vary depending on the type of CT procedure, patient size, CT system, and operating technique.[28–30]

PHYSIOLOGIC AND VARIANT FLUORODEOXYGLUCOSE DISTRIBUTION IN CHILDREN

Thymus and bone growth centers may show increased FDG uptake and is specific for children.[31,32] Increased FDG uptake has been encountered in the brain (mainly the subcortical gray matter)[27]; salivary glands; myocardium; renal pelves; ureters; and bladder. There is mild uptake of liver, spleen, and bone marrow. Occasionally, FDG uptake may also be noted in the thyroid gland and vocal cords.[33–35] Following chemotherapy, diffuse increased FDG uptake has been noted in bone marrow, in spleen, and occasionally in the thymus.[36–38] Increased FDG activity in the breast of a teenage girl or in the testicle of a teenage boy is frequent and should be regarded as normal variant. In addition, brown fat activity in pediatric population is frequently more prevalent and more intense.

GASTROINTESTINAL LYMPHOMA

Non-Hodgkin's lymphoma accounts for about 60% of all lymphomas and 10% of childhood malignancies.[39] Primary extranodal lymphoma represents 25% of the non-Hodgkin's lymphoma incidence in the United States. Approximately 50% of extranodal lymphoma occur in the gastrointestinal tract.[40,41] In the pediatric group, small and large intestines are the most common locations of involvement (**Fig. 1**). Every extranodal site has special clinical characteristics and management.[42] Hodgkin's disease, a malignant process of the lymphoreticular system, constitutes 6% of childhood cancers.[39] Approximately 30% of children with Hodgkin's disease have the propensity of extranodal spread including liver and spleen.[43] Studies show that most extranodal lymphomas arise from lymphoid cells of lineage different from those of the lymph nodes and spleen.[44,45] The alternative lymphoid system is known as mucosa-associated lymphoid tissue. Mucosa-associated lymphoid tissue lymphocytes have specific receptors that allow homing to extranodal tissues.[46] The homing capacity of mucosa-associated lymphoid tissue lymphocytes can explain some of the extranodal spread pattern.[47] Immunophenotype of mucosa-associated lymphoid tissue lymphomas helps distinguish them from other neoplastic proliferations of small lymphoid cells. Mucosa-associated lymphoid tissue lymphocytes are positive for clonal surface Ig and pan B-cell antigens (CD22, CD20, and CD19), but negative for both CD5 and for CD10.[48,49] The prognosis of childhood lymphoma has improved with survival rate of about 90%.[39]

FDG-PET and PET-CT proved to be useful for detection, staging, restaging, monitoring therapy response, and evaluation of recurrence in patients with lymphoma.[9,50–54] The routine application of PET imaging in pediatric oncology, however, has not been fully established.[55]

CT remains the most commonly used modality in management of patients with lymphomas.[56–58] CT interpretation depends on the size and shape of lesions, however, which takes time to be detectable. Furthermore, CT may not differentiate between fibrosis-necrosis and residual disease after therapy.[59–61] For many years, gallium scintigraphy has been the functional imaging modality for high-grade non-Hodgkin's lymphoma at the time of diagnosis and in evaluation of response to treatment that may solve some CT challenging cases.[33,62] Gallium, however, has some drawbacks. It has low sensitivity and specificity for infradiaphragmatic disease because of physiologic uptake of gallium in the abdomen. Because of low resolution, it is difficult to evaluate intermediate and low-grade lymphomas. Moreover, a long time interval between injection and scanning (3 days) is required to clear the background activity.[33]

PET imaging has features that make it preferable to gallium scintigraphy: a shorter interval between

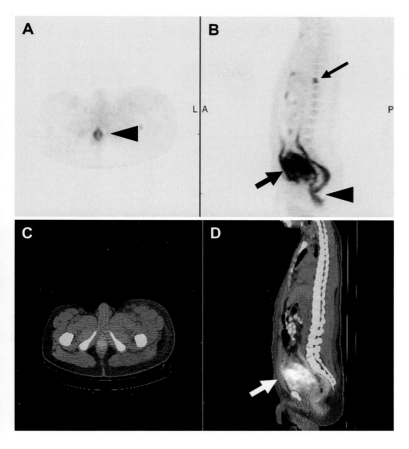

Fig. 1. Lymphoma with bowel involvement FDG-PET (*upper row L-R, A, B*) and fused PET-CT (*lower row*) axial (*left side, C*) and sagittal (*right side, D*) images of an 18-year-old man with Burkitt's lymphoma. Sagittal images show an increased FDG uptake in a large pelvic mass (*short arrows*). Diffuse increased activity involving the rectal wall, seen on axial and sagittal images (*arrowhead*). There is also bone marrow involvement (*long arrow*).

injection to imaging time allowing completion of the study in a few hours, more favorable dosimetry, and better image quality and resolution.[63] In addition, combination of PET with CT improves the diagnostic potential through evaluating both metabolic and structural data in synergistic manner.[7]

FDG-PET revealed high sensitivity and specificity in patients with lymphoma. Mody and colleagues[64] demonstrated sensitivity and specificity of 90% and 88% in children with non-Hodgkin's lymphoma, respectively. A sensitivity of 78% and specificity of 89% have been reported by Hernandez-Pampaloni and colleagues.[12] Furth and coworkers[65] showed 96% accuracy for FDG-PET in detecting extranodal disease in 33 children with Hodgkin's disease. Another study that included Hodgkin's lymphoma patients by Hutchings and colleagues[66] revealed sensitivity and specificity of PET-CT to be 97.7% and 100%, respectively, for abdominal and pelvic disease. In the initial staging, FDG-PET has been found to change disease stage in 10% to 23% of children with lymphoma.[67–70] In several studies, PET imaging revealed disease sites that had not been detected by regular staging methods with

potential upstaging of disease. Miller and colleagues[71] reported that in a series of 31 children diagnosed with lymphoma, FDG-PET-CT upstaged 22.6% of cases by detecting nodal and extranodal disease overlooked on a diagnostic CT imaging. In the same study,[71] PET-CT has downstaged 9.6% of cases by excluding disease in nonspecific lesions. False-positive FDG-PET results may occur in inflammatory and reactive conditions of the gastrointestinal tract, some physiologic uptake of bowel, and after recent surgery.[72] Although not common, transient inflammatory changes as a reaction to therapy may occur following radiation or chemotherapy.[73] False-negative results may occur with small or flat mucosal lesions, however, blurring by movement and the variable metabolic contrast of different tissues.[65] FDG activity in the known lesions following chemotherapy has become a crucial factor in assessing the efficacy of the therapy (**Fig. 2**).

HEPATIC TUMORS

Primary tumors of the liver account for 1% of malignancies in children, with more than 65% of these

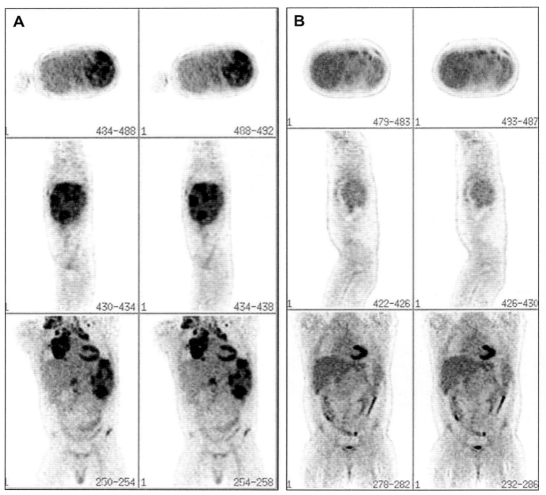

Fig. 2. Pretreatment (*A*) and posttreatment (*B*) FDG-PET images of a teenage boy with Hodgkin's lymphoma. There is interval resolution of multiple hypermetabolic lesions including lymphomatous spleen and lymphadenopathy involving supraclavicular, mediastinal including large hilar lesion, and celiac nodes. The patient received localized radiation to the right hilar mass and chemotherapy.

malignancies being hepatoblastomas and most of the remainder hepatocellular carcinomas.[74] Rare hepatic malignancies include angiosarcoma, malignant germ cell tumor, rhabdomyosarcoma of the liver, and undifferentiated sarcoma. Furthermore, other childhood malignancies can metastasize to the liver.[74]

HEPATOBLASTOMA

Hepatoblastoma is an embryonal tumor, and 90% of cases are manifest by the age of 4 years.[76,77] Alpha fetoprotein level is elevated in 90% of children with hepatoblastoma and the remaining 10% of cases tend to be more aggressive.[78,79] Hepatoblastoma usually presents as large multinodular masses. They disseminate to lungs and contiguous tissues.[74] Cure from hepatoblastoma is defined as a complete gross resection of the primary tumor. Resection at diagnosis, whenever possible, is adapted by many clinicians.[80] Alternatively, neoadjuvant chemotherapy is advised for all patients with the argument that chemotherapy renders most tumors smaller, better demarcated, and likely to be completely resected. Furthermore, liver transplantation has shown to be a good option in children with unresectable hepatoblastoma and without demonstrable metastatic disease after neoadjuvant chemotherapy.[68,81,82]

Hepatoblastoma tends to have increased glycolytic activity. This allows FDG-PET imaging to assess the extent of disease, the presence of metastasis, and response to therapy. In five patients with suspected hepatoblastoma, Mody and colleagues[64] reported increased FDG uptake in all the cases. One case, however, turned out to be necrotizing granuloma at surgery. The same case was positive on CT with high alpha fetoprotein. Most of the available reports in the literature have focused on the usefulness of PET in the detection of recurrence of hepatoblastoma. FDG-PET successfully located the site of recurrence in a series of three patients with recurrent hepatoblastoma in a study by Philip and colleagues.[83] Figarola and colleagues[84] presented a single case where FDG-PET detected recurrent hepatoblastoma that has not been reported with other imaging modalities. Interestingly, Sironi and colleagues[85] reported FDG-PET detection of a recurrent hepatoblastoma in a transplanted liver. FDG-PET revealed multiple areas of focal FDG accumulation in the liver and peritoneum, all of them confirmed on pathology. In contrast, other imaging modalities suggested a single hepatic lesion where additional liver lesions and peritoneal implants were not detected. Wong and colleagues,[86] however, in a series of 10 children who underwent FDG-PET as part of their posttherapy evaluation, reported that three patients had PET findings suggestive of recurrent hepatoblastoma and two of them had elevated alpha fetoprotein. The three cases were false-positives. Negative FDG-PET scans support absence of detectable recurrence. Positive scans, however, should be carefully interpreted and correlated with other clinical findings.

OTHER HEPATIC MALIGNANCY

Hepatocellular carcinoma can occur in adolescents and is mostly associated with hepatitis B or C infections.[75] Pediatric hepatocellular carcinoma usually expresses elevated serum levels of alpha fetoprotein. Abnormal liver function tests, such as alanine aminotransferase, total bilirubin, albumin, and alkaline phosphatase, are uncommon, however, in patients with pediatric liver tumors.[87] Complete resection of this tumor is possible in 30% to 40% of cases. The prognosis is poor; only 30% of children are long-term survivors.[75] Currently, there is no publication specific for FDG-PET in pediatric hepatocellular carcinoma. Evaluation of FDG-PET in hepatocellular carcinoma in adults with cirrhosis revealed low sensitivity with better results in the detection of extrahepatic metastases.[88-93] Detection of hepatocellular carcinoma in pediatric patients without cirrhosis, however, seems more promising (**Fig. 3**).

Hepatic metastases in children, although rare, may occur from neuroblastoma, Wilms' tumor, osteogenic sarcoma, malignant gastric epithelial tumor, and desmoplastic small round cell tumor.[3-5] Shulkin and colleagues[94] reported a case of hepatic sarcoma that showed intense FDG uptake. A definite role of FDG-PET in pediatric liver metastases has not been fully established. The authors' experience showed, however, that FDG-PET had high sensitivity and specificity for metastatic liver lesions in pediatric patients (**Fig. 4**), as has been demonstrated in adults.[95-97]

PANCREATIC TUMORS

Pancreatic tumors can be of endocrine or nonendocrine origin. Endocrine tumors include insulinomas and gastrinomas. Insulinomas lead to congenital hyperinsulinism, which is the most common cause of persistent hypoglycemia in infancy.[98] Hypoglycemia accompanied by high insulin level or gastric ulcers (Zollinger-Ellison syndrome) indicates the possibility of a pancreatic tumor.[99] When there is resistance to medical treatment attempts, surgical intervention is the treatment of choice. If the primary tumor cannot be located or if it has metastasized, however, cure may not be possible.[100] Unsuccessful and inadequate control of hypoglycemia may result in adverse neurologic damage.[101,102]

Pancreatoblastomas, pancreatic adenocarcinomas, cystadenomas, and rhabdomyosarcomas are nonendocrine tumors and are rarely encountered. Resection, when possible, can be curative. Presurgical chemotherapy may be considered for lesions that are not primarily respectable.[103-107]

Hyperinsulinism lesions can be focal or diffuse[108,109]; these two entities are clinically indistinguishable.[110-112] Focal hyperinsulinism represents about half of the cases.[113] Pathologically, the pancreatic β-cells are gathered in a focal adenoma. Diffuse hyperinsulinism corresponds to disseminated β-cells in the whole pancreas, however, showing enlarged abnormal nuclei.[114,115] Differentiation between focal and diffuse forms and the precise localization of a focal lesion in congenital hyperinsulinism is critical when planning surgery.[116] Focal hyperinsulinism is cured by selective resection of the lesion, whereas diffuse hyperinsulinism requires subtotal pancreatectomy, with severe iatrogenic diabetes as a consequence.[117-119]

L-3,4-Dihydroxyphenylalanine (L-dopa) is a precursor of catecholamines that is converted to dopamine by aromatic amino acid decarboxylase.[120] Pancreatic islets have been shown to take up L-dopa and convert it to dopamine.[121-123] Fluorine-18- fluoro-L-dopa (F-dopa) PET has been

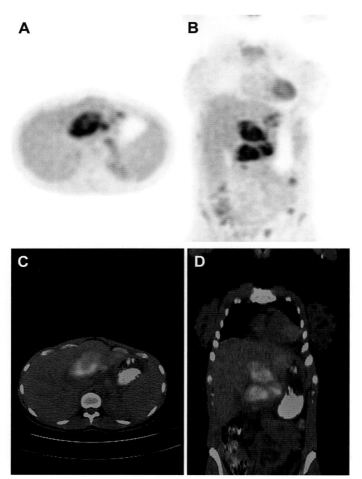

Fig. 3. FDG-PET (*upper row, A, B*) and fused PET-CT (*lower row, C, D*) images of a young woman with abdominal pain. Axial (*left side, A, C*) and coronal (*right side, B, D*) images demonstrate FDG avid malignancy in the left hepatic lobe and para-aortic nodes. The liver lesion was proved to be fibrolamellar hepatocellular carcinoma by histopathologic examination.

proved to be effective, with highly promising results, in distinguishing between focal and diffuse disease (**Fig. 5**) and with histopathology confirmation.[115,124–126] Mohnike and colleagues[127] in a consensus paper reported a sensitivity and specificity of 94% and 100% for F-dopa PET, respectively. Hardy and colleagues[128] analyzed 50 infants with hyperinsulinism and unresponsive to medical therapy. F-dopa PET correctly differentiated focal and diffuse disease in 88% of cases and accurately identified 75% of cases with focal disease. Similar findings had been noted by Ribeiro and colleagues.[124] F-dopa PET results had been confirmed by histopathology in 87.5% of cases. Barthlen and colleagues[116] investigated 10 children with signs of congenital hyperinsulinism and a focal F-dopa uptake in the pancreas. In nine children, a limited resection of the pancreas corresponding to site of F-dopa uptake was curative. The results of F-dopa PET seem to be better than arterial calcium stimulation with hepatic vein insulin sampling and transhepatic portal venous insulin

sampling in differentiating focal from diffuse disease of the pancreas and in identifying the location of the focal lesion.[113,129] Currently, the integrated PET-CT method enables both exact anatomic and functional description of the pancreatic focus.[116] Drug interference with F-dopa metabolism should be considered. It has been noted that somatostatin and diazoxide may not interfere with F-dopa. Glucagon has been known to interfere with F-dopa uptake, however, and it is recommended to stop it 2 days before F-dopa PET.[124] The effect of carbidopa on the detection of focal form of congenital hyperinsulinism has not been established at this time.

LIMITATIONS AND PITFALLS

The use of PET-CT and other imaging modalities in the management of pediatric malignancies raises concerns about radiation exposure in children. There is higher risk of radiation-induced malignancies in children relative to adults.[130] It is important

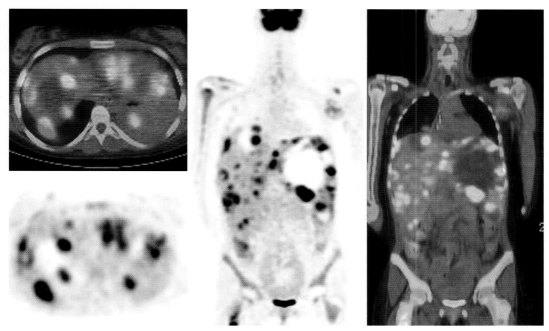

Fig. 4. An 18-year-old woman with melanoma. FDG PET-CT demonstrated multiple metastases in the liver and spleen. There is also bone and bone marrow involvement. Two large liver cysts are seen in the dome of the liver and left hepatic lobe.

to keep radiation exposure as low as is reasonably achievable (ALARA principle).[131,132]

Intravenous contrast, if indicated, may cause artifacts related to attenuation correction.[133] Oral contrast may affect semiquantitative measures including standardized uptake value.[134–136] Furthermore, standardized uptake value in pediatric patients can be different from that in adult patients because of the body changes that occur during childhood. Standardized uptake value calculation based on body surface area seems to be more uniform in pediatric patients.[137]

Transient inflammatory changes as a reaction to radiation and, less commonly, chemotherapy may lead to false-positive PET results. A time window between completion of therapy and performance of PET imaging is advised. It is recommended to wait 3, and preferably 6 to 8, weeks after chemotherapy, and 8 to 12 weeks after radiation therapy.[72,138]

SUMMARY

PET and PET-CT are increasingly used in pediatric oncology.[33] The available literature showed that PET may provide additional information that can significantly help in the diagnosis, staging, and management guidelines. Furthermore, PET may have great potential in predicting the response to treatment in early stage of therapy.[11,12,53,55,89,116,139,140] In extranodal lymphoma, FDG-PET seems to be an important tool

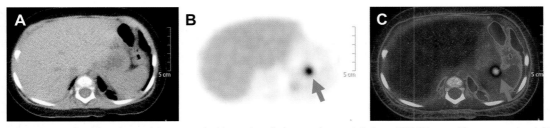

Fig. 5. A 7-month-old patient with congenital hyperinsulinism underwent F-dopa PET-CT scan. The noncontrast CT image (A) was unremarkable. The F-dopa PET image (B), however, revealed a focal activity (arrow) corresponding to the end of the tail of the pancreas on the fused PET-CT image (C). Surgical pathology confirmed the focal form of congenital hyperinsulinism.

in the initial diagnosis and follow-up after therapy.[53,54,66] Furthermore, FDG-PET revealed promising results in cases with hepatoblastoma, especially when recurrence is evaluated.[78,79] PET using F-dopa has been found to be a highly promising and noninvasive method allowing differentiation between focal and diffuse disease in cases with congenital hyperinsulinism.[127,128]

The role of PET imaging in other childhood gastrointestinal malignancies is not well established. Further trials and studies are encouraged to delineate and identify the role of PET in pediatric oncology.

REFERENCES

1. Ries LAG, Krapcho M, Stinchcomb DG, et al, editors. SEER Cancer Statistics Review, 1975–2005, National Cancer Institute. Bethesda (MD), Available at: http://seer.cancer.gov/csr/1975_2005/. Accessed November 2007 SEER data submission, posted to the SEER web site, 2008.
2. Jemal A, Siegel R, Ward E, et al. Cancer statistics, 2008. CA Cancer J Clin 2008;58(2):71–96.
3. Fuchs J, Szavay P, Luithle T, et al. Surgical implications for liver metastases in nephroblastoma–data from the SIOP/GPOH study. Surg Oncol 2008; 17:33–40.
4. Szavay P, Luithle T, Graf N, et al. Primary hepatic metastases in nephroblastoma: a report of the SIOP/GPOH Study. J Pediatr Surg 2006;41(1): 168–72 [discussion 168–72].
5. Su WT, Rutigliano DN, Gholizadeh M, et al. Hepatic metastasectomy in children. Cancer 2007;109(10): 2089–92.
6. Kadan-Lottick NS. Epidemiology of Childhood and Adolescent Cancer. In: Kliegman R, Jenson HB, Behrman RE, Stanton Bonita F, eds. Nelson textbook of pediatrics. Eighteenth Edition ed. Philadelphia, PA: Saunders Elsevier, 2007.
7. Von Schulthess GK, Hany TF. Imaging and PET-PET/CT imaging. J Radiol 2008;89(3 Pt 2):438–47 quiz 448.
8. Kurmasheva RT, Houghton PJ. Pediatric oncology. Curr Opin Chem Biol 2007;11(4):424–32.
9. Castell F, Cook GJ. Quantitative techniques in 18FDG PET scanning in oncology. Br J Cancer 2008;98(10):1597–601.
10. Maldonado A, Gonzalez-Alenda FJ, Alonso M, et al. PET-CT in clinical oncology. Clin Transl Oncol 2007;9(8):494–505.
11. Al-Nahhas A, Win Z, Singh A, et al. The role of 18F-FDG PET in oncology: clinical and resource implications. Nucl Med Rev Cent East Eur 2006;9(1):1–5.
12. Hernandez-Pampaloni M, Takalkar A, Yu JQ, et al. F-18 FDG-PET imaging and correlation with CT in staging and follow-up of pediatric lymphomas. Pediatr Radiol 2006;36(6):524–31.
13. Cermik TF, Mavi A, Basu S, et al. Impact of FDG PET on the preoperative staging of newly diagnosed breast cancer. Eur J Nucl Med Mol Imaging 2008;35(3):475–83.
14. Hustinx R, Benard F, Alavi A. Whole-body FDG-PET imaging in the management of patients with cancer. Semin Nucl Med 2002;32(1):35–46.
15. Zhang Y, Xiu Y, Zhuang H, et al. Follow-up FDG PET in the evaluation of unexplained focal activity in the abdomen. Clin Nucl Med 2008;33(1): 19–22.
16. Xiu Y, Bhutani C, Dhurairaj T, et al. Dual-time point FDG PET imaging in the evaluation of pulmonary nodules with minimally increased metabolic activity. Clin Nucl Med 2007;32(2):101–5.
17. Collins CD. PET/CT in oncology: for which tumours is it the reference standard? Cancer Imaging 2007; 7(Spec No A):S77–87.
18. Roca I, Simo M, Sabado C, et al. PET/CT in paediatrics: it is time to increase its use! Eur J Nucl Med Mol Imaging 2007;34(5):628–9.
19. Franzius C, Juergens KU, Schober O. Is PET/CT necessary in paediatric oncology? For. Eur J Nucl Med Mol Imaging 2006;33(8):960–5.
20. Stauss J, Franzius C, Pfluger T, et al. Guidelines for (18)F-FDG PET and PET-CT imaging in paediatric oncology. Eur J Nucl Med Mol Imaging 2008; 33(8):1581–8.
21. Gordon I. Issues surrounding preparation, information and handling the child and parent in nuclear medicine. J Nucl Med 1998;39(3):490–4.
22. Shulkin BL. PET imaging in pediatric oncology. Pediatr Radiol 2004;34(3):199–204.
23. Mandell GA, Cooper JA, Majd M, et al. Procedure guideline for pediatric sedation in nuclear medicine. Society of Nuclear Medicine. J Nucl Med 1997;38(10):1640–3.
24. American Academy of Pediatrics Committee on Drugs: Guidelines for monitoring and management of pediatric patients during and after sedation for diagnostic and therapeutic procedures. Pediatrics 1992;89(6 Pt 1):1110–5.
25. Shulkin BL. PET applications in pediatrics. Q J Nucl Med 1997;41(4):281–91.
26. Schelbert HR, Hoh CK, Royal HD, et al. Procedure guideline for tumor imaging using fluorine-18-FDG. Society of Nuclear Medicine. J Nucl Med 1998; 39(7):1302–5.
27. Ruotsalainen U, Suhonen-Polvi H, Eronen E, et al. Estimated radiation dose to the newborn in FDG-PET studies. J Nucl Med 1996;37(2):387–93.
28. Bertell R, Ehrle LH, Schmitz-Feuerhake I. Pediatric CT research elevates public health concerns: low-dose radiation issues are highly politicized. Int J Health Serv 2007;37(3):419–39.

29. Gelfand MJ, Lemen LC. PET/CT and SPECT/CT dosimetry in children: the challenge to the pediatric imager. Semin Nucl Med 2007;37(5):391–8.

30. Hidajat N, Maurer J, Schroder RJ, et al. Relationships between physical dose quantities and patient dose in CT. Br J Radiol 1999;72(858):556–61.

31. Weinblatt ME, Zanzi I, Belakhlef A, et al. False-positive FDG-PET imaging of the thymus of a child with Hodgkin's disease. J Nucl Med 1997;38(6):888–90.

32. Patel PM, Alibazoglu H, Ali A, et al. Normal thymic uptake of FDG on PET imaging. Clin Nucl Med 1996;21(10):772–5.

33. Jadvar H, Alavi A, Mavi A, et al. PET in pediatric diseases. Radiol Clin North Am 2005;43(1):135–52.

34. Delbeke D. Oncological applications of FDG PET imaging: brain tumors, colorectal cancer, lymphoma and melanoma. J Nucl Med 1999;40(4):591–603.

35. El-Haddad G, Alavi A, Mavi A, et al. Normal variants in [18F]-fluorodeoxyglucose PET imaging. Radiol Clin North Am 2004;42(6):1063–181.

36. Siehr DJ. Studies on the cell wall of Schizophyllum commune. Permethylation and enzymic hydrolysis. Can J Biochem 1976;54(2):130–6.

37. Hollinger EF, Alibazoglu H, Ali A, et al. Hematopoietic cytokine-mediated FDG uptake simulates the appearance of diffuse metastatic disease on whole-body PET imaging. Clin Nucl Med 1998;23(2):93–8.

38. Brink I, Reinhardt MJ, Hoegerle S, et al. Increased metabolic activity in the thymus gland studied with 18F-FDG PET: age dependency and frequency after chemotherapy. J Nucl Med 2001;42(4):591–5.

39. Cairo MS, Bradley MB, et al. Lymphoma. In: Kliegman R, editor. Nelson textbook of pediatrics. Philadelphia: Saunders Elsevier; 2007.

40. Ford E. Gastrointestinal tumors. In: Andrassy R, editor. Pediatric surgical oncology. Philadelphia: WB Saunders Co; 1998. p. 289–304.

41. Ferry JA. Extranodal lymphoma. Arch Pathol Lab Med 2008;132(4):565–78.

42. Aisenberg A. Malignant lymphoma: biology, natural history and treatment. Philadelphia: Lea & Feibiger; 1991.

43. Oguz A, Karadeniz C, Okur FV, et al. Prognostic factors and treatment outcome in childhood Hodgkin disease. Pediatr Blood Cancer 2005;45(5):670–5.

44. Bienenstock J, Befus AD. Mucosal immunology. Immunology 1980;41(2):249–70.

45. Isaacson PG, Spencer J. Malignant lymphoma of mucosa-associated lymphoid tissue. Histopathology 1987;11(5):445–62.

46. Carbone PP, Kaplan HS, Musshoff K, et al. Report of the Committee on Hodgkin's Disease Staging Classification. Cancer Res 1971;31(11):1860–1.

47. Aisenberg AC. Coherent view of non-Hodgkin's lymphoma. J Clin Oncol 1995;13(10):2656–75.

48. Harris NL, Jaffe ES, Stein H, et al. A revised European-American classification of lymphoid neoplasms: a proposal from the International Lymphoma Study Group. Blood 1994;84(5):1361–92.

49. Shivdasani RA, Hess JL, Skarin AT, et al. Intermediate lymphocytic lymphoma: clinical and pathologic features of a recently characterized subtype of non-Hodgkin's lymphoma. J Clin Oncol 1993;11(4):802–11.

50. Enomoto K, Hamada K, Inohara H, et al. Mucosa-associated lymphoid tissue lymphoma studied with FDG-PET: a comparison with CT and endoscopic findings. Ann Nucl Med 2008;22(4):261–7.

51. Takahashi T, Minato M, Tsukuda H, et al. Successful treatment of intravascular large B-cell lymphoma diagnosed by bone marrow biopsy and FDG-PET scan. Intern Med 2008;47(10):975–9.

52. Bural GG, Shriaknthan S, Houseni M, et al. FDG-PET is useful in staging and follow-up of primary uterine cervical lymphoma. Clin Nucl Med 2007;32(9):748–50.

53. Ambrosini V, Rubello D, Castellucci P, et al. Diagnostic role of 18F-FDG PET in gastric MALT lymphoma. Nucl Med Rev Cent East Eur 2006;9(1):37–40.

54. Kasamon YL, Wahl RL. FDG PET and risk-adapted therapy in Hodgkin's and non-Hodgkin's lymphoma. Curr Opin Oncol 2008;20(2):206–19.

55. Tatsumi M, Miller JH, Wahl RL. 18F-FDG PET/CT in evaluating non-CNS pediatric malignancies. J Nucl Med 2007;48(12):1923–31.

56. Yu RS, Zhang WM, Liu YQ. CT diagnosis of 52 patients with lymphoma in abdominal lymph nodes. World J Gastroenterol 2006;12(48):7869–73.

57. Lupescu IG, Grasu M, Goldis G, et al. Computer tomographic evaluation of digestive tract non-Hodgkin lymphomas. J Gastrointestin Liver Dis 2007;16(3):315–9.

58. Pelosi E, Pregno P, Penna D, et al. Role of whole-body [(18)F] fluorodeoxyglucose positron emission tomography/computed tomography (FDG-PET/CT) and conventional techniques in the staging of patients with Hodgkin and aggressive non Hodgkin lymphoma. Torino: Radiol Med; 2008.

59. Zinzani PL, Magagnoli M, Chierichetti F, et al. The role of positron emission tomography (PET) in the management of lymphoma patients. Ann Oncol 1999;10(10):1181–4.

60. Gollub MJ, Hong R, Sarasohn DM, et al. Limitations of CT during PET/CT. J Nucl Med 2007;48(10):1583–91.

61. Pelosi E, Penna D, Deandreis D, et al. FDG-PET in the detection of bone marrow disease in Hodgkin's disease and aggressive non-Hodgkin's lymphoma and its impact on clinical management. Q J Nucl Med Mol Imaging 2008;52(1):9–16.

62. Ballani NS, Khan HA, Al-Mohannadi SH, et al. Role of serial quantitative gallium-67 tumor uptake in assessing response rates for chemotherapy in lymphoma patients. Nucl Med Commun 2008;29(6): 527–34.

63. Seam P, Juweid ME, Cheson BD. The role of FDG-PET scans in patients with lymphoma. Blood 2007; 110(10):3507–16.

64. Mody RJ, Bui C, Hutchinson RJ, et al. Comparison of (18)F flurodeoxyglucose PET with Ga-67 scintigraphy and conventional imaging modalities in pediatric lymphoma. Leuk Lymphoma 2007;48(4): 699–707.

65. Furth C, Denecke T, Steffen I, et al. Correlative imaging strategies implementing CT, MRI, and PET for staging of childhood Hodgkin disease. J Pediatr Hematol Oncol 2006;28(8):501–12.

66. Hutchings M, Loft A, Hansen M, et al. Position emission tomography with or without computed tomography in the primary staging of Hodgkin's lymphoma. Haematologica 2006;91(4):482–9.

67. Amthauer H, Furth C, Denecke T, et al. FDG-PET in 10 children with non-Hodgkin's lymphoma: initial experience in staging and follow-up. Klin Padiatr 2005;217(6):327–33.

68. Depas G, De Barsy C, Jerusalem G, et al. 18F-FDG PET in children with lymphomas. Eur J Nucl Med Mol Imaging 2005;32(1):31–8.

69. Kabickova E, Sumerauer D, Cumlivska E, et al. Comparison of 18F-FDG-PET and standard procedures for the pretreatment staging of children and adolescents with Hodgkin's disease. Eur J Nucl Med Mol Imaging 2006;33(9):1025–31.

70. Montravers F, McNamara D, Landman-Parker J, et al. [(18)F]FDG in childhood lymphoma: clinical utility and impact on management. Eur J Nucl Med Mol Imaging 2002;29(9):1155–65.

71. Miller E, Metser U, Avrahami G, et al. Role of 18F-FDG PET/CT in staging and follow-up of lymphoma in pediatric and young adult patients. J Comput Assist Tomogr 2006;30(4):689–94.

72. Beker DB, Berrak SG, Canpolat C, et al. False positivity of FDG-PET/CT in a child with Hodgkin disease. Pediatr Blood Cancer 2008;50(4):881–3.

73. Brepoels L, Stroobants S. Is [(18)F]fluorodeoxyglucose positron emission tomography the ultimate tool for response and prognosis assessment? Hematol Oncol Clin North Am 2007;21(5):855–69.

74. Meyers RL. Tumors of the liver in children. Surg Oncol 2007;16(3):195–203.

75. Herzog CE, et al. Neoplasms of the liver. In: Kliegman R, editor. Nelson textbook of pediatrics. Philadelphia: Saunders Elsevier 2007.

76. Ansell P, Mitchell CD, Roman E, et al. Relationships between perinatal and maternal characteristics and hepatoblastoma: a report from the UKCCS. Eur J Cancer 2005;41(5):741–8.

77. Oue T, Kubota A, Okuyama H, et al. Hepatoblastoma in children of extremely low birth weight: a report from a single perinatal center. J Pediatr Surg 2003;38(1):134–7 [discussion 134–7].

78. Malogolowkin MH, Katzenstein HM, Krailo M, et al. Redefining the role of doxorubicin for the treatment of children with hepatoblastoma. J Clin Oncol 2008; 26(14):2379–83.

79. Meyers RL, Katzenstein HM, Malogolowkin MH. Predictive value of staging systems in hepatoblastoma. J Clin Oncol 2007;25(6):737 author reply 737–8.

80. von Schweinitz D, Hecker H, Schmidt-von-Arndt G, et al. Prognostic factors and staging systems in childhood hepatoblastoma. Int J Cancer 1997; 74(6):593–9.

81. Czauderna P, Otte JB, Roebuck DJ, et al. Surgical treatment of hepatoblastoma in children. Pediatr Radiol 2006;36(3):187–91.

82. Czauderna P, Otte JB, Aronson DC, et al. Guidelines for surgical treatment of hepatoblastoma in the modern era: recommendations from the Childhood Liver Tumour Strategy Group of the International Society of Paediatric Oncology (SIOPEL). Eur J Cancer 2005;41(7):1031–6.

83. Philip I, Shun A, McCowage G, et al. Positron emission tomography in recurrent hepatoblastoma. Pediatr Surg Int 2005;21(5):341–5.

84. Figarola MS, McQuiston SA, Wilson F, et al. Recurrent hepatoblastoma with localization by PET-CT. Pediatr Radiol 2005;35(12):1254–8.

85. Sironi S, Messa C, Cistaro A, et al. Recurrent hepatoblastoma in orthotopic transplanted liver: detection with FDG positron emission tomography. AJR Am J Roentgenol 2004;182(5):1214–6.

86. Wong KK, Lan LC, Lin SC, et al. The use of positron emission tomography in detecting hepatoblastoma recurrence–a cautionary tale. J Pediatr Surg 2004; 39(12):1779–81.

87. Wang JD, Chang TK, Chen HC, et al. Pediatric liver tumors: initial presentation, image finding and outcome. Pediatr Int 2007;49(4):491–6.

88. He YX, Guo QY. Clinical applications and advances of positron emission tomography with fluorine-18-fluorodeoxyglucose (18F-FDG) in the diagnosis of liver neoplasms. Postgrad Med J 2008;84(991): 246–51.

89. Ho CL, Chen S, Yeung DW, et al. Dual-tracer PET/CT imaging in evaluation of metastatic hepatocellular carcinoma. J Nucl Med 2007;48(6):902–9.

90. Shin JA, Park JW, An M, et al [Diagnostic accuracy of 18F-FDG positron emission tomography for evaluation of hepatocellular carcinoma]. Korean J Hepatol 2006;12(4):546–52.

91. Sun L, Guan YS, Pan WM, et al. Positron emission tomography/computer tomography in guidance of extrahepatic hepatocellular carcinoma metastasis management. World J Gastroenterol 2007;13(40): 5413–5.

92. Talbot JN, Gutman F, Fartoux L, et al. PET/CT in patients with hepatocellular carcinoma using [(18)F]fluorocholine: preliminary comparison with [(18)F]FDG PET/CT. Eur J Nucl Med Mol Imaging 2006;33(11):1285–9.

93. Yoon KT, Kim JK, Kim do Y, et al. Role of 18F-fluorodeoxyglucose positron emission tomography in detecting extrahepatic metastasis in pretreatment staging of hepatocellular carcinoma. Oncology 2007;72(Suppl 1):104–10.

94. Shulkin BL, Mitchell DS, Ungar DR, et al. Neoplasms in a pediatric population: 2-[F-18]-fluoro-2-deoxy-D-glucose PET studies. Radiology 1995; 194(2):495–500.

95. Kong G, Jackson C, Koh DM, et al. The use of (18)F-FDG PET/CT in colorectal liver metastases-comparison with CT and liver MRI. Eur J Nucl Med Mol Imaging 2008;35(7):1323–9.

96. Huguet EL, Old S, Praseedom RK, et al. F18-FDG-PET evaluation of patients for resection of colorectal liver metastases. Hepatogastroenterology 2007;54(78):1667–71.

97. Zhuang H, Sinha P, Pourdehnad M, et al. The role of positron emission tomography with fluorine-18-deoxyglucose in identifying colorectal cancer metastases to liver. Nucl Med Commun 2000;21(9): 793–8.

98. Kloppel G, Anlauf M. Gastrinoma: morphological aspects. Wien Klin Wochenschr 2007;119(19-20): 579–84.

99. Pellicano R, De Angelis C, Resegotti A, et al. Zollinger-Ellison syndrome in 2006: concepts from a clinical point of view. Panminerva Med 2006;48(1): 33–40.

100. Akerstrom G, Hellman P. Surgery on neuroendocrine tumours. Best Pract Res Clin Endocrinol Metab 2007;21(1):87–109.

101. Dekelbab BH, Sperling MA. Recent advances in hyperinsulinemic hypoglycemia of infancy. Acta Paediatr 2006;95(10):1157–64.

102. Menni F, de Lonlay P, Sevin C, et al. Neurologic outcomes of 90 neonates and infants with persistent hyperinsulinemic hypoglycemia. Pediatrics 2001; 107(3):476–9.

103. Barenboim-Stapleton L, Yang X, Tsokos M, et al. Pediatric pancreatoblastoma: histopathologic and cytogenetic characterization of tumor and derived cell line. Cancer Genet Cytogenet 2005;157(2): 109–17.

104. Hasegawa Y, Ishida Y, Kato K, et al. Pancreatoblastoma: a case report with special emphasis on squamoid corpuscles with optically clear nuclei rich in biotin. Acta Cytol 2003;47(4):679–84.

105. Kletter GB, Sweetser DA, Wallace SF, et al. Adrenocorticotropin-secreting pancreatoblastoma. J Pediatr Endocrinol Metab 2007;20(5):639–42.

106. Palladino AA, Bennett MJ, Stanley CA. Hyperinsulinism in infancy and childhood: when an insulin level is not always enough. Clin Chem 2008; 54(2):256–63.

107. Sugai M, Kimura N, Umehara M, et al. A case of pancreatoblastoma prenatally diagnosed as intraperitoneal cyst. Pediatr Surg Int 2006;22(10): 845–7.

108. Goossens A, Gepts W, Saudubray JM, et al. Diffuse and focal nesidioblastosis: a clinicopathological study of 24 patients with persistent neonatal hyperinsulinemic hypoglycemia. Am J Surg Pathol 1989; 13(9):766–75.

109. Rahier J, Falt K, Muntefering H, et al. The basic structural lesion of persistent neonatal hypoglycaemia with hyperinsulinism: deficiency of pancreatic D cells or hyperactivity of B cells? Diabetologia 1984;26(4):282–9.

110. de Lonlay P, Fournet JC, Rahier J, et al. Somatic deletion of the imprinted 11p15 region in sporadic persistent hyperinsulinemic hypoglycemia of infancy is specific of focal adenomatous hyperplasia and endorses partial pancreatectomy. J Clin Invest 1997;100(4):802–7.

111. Nestorowicz A, Wilson BA, Schoor KP, et al. Mutations in the sulonylurea receptor gene are associated with familial hyperinsulinism in Ashkenazi Jews. Hum Mol Genet 1996;5(11):1813–22.

112. Thomas PM, Cote GJ, Wohllk N, et al. Mutations in the sulfonylurea receptor gene in familial persistent hyperinsulinemic hypoglycemia of infancy. Science 1995;268(5209):426–9.

113. de Lonlay-Debeney P, Poggi-Travert F, Fournet JC, et al. Clinical features of 52 neonates with hyperinsulinism. N Engl J Med 1999;340(15):1169–75.

114. Sempoux C, Guiot Y, Lefevre A, et al. Neonatal hyperinsulinemic hypoglycemia: heterogeneity of the syndrome and keys for differential diagnosis. J Clin Endocrinol Metab 1998;83(5):1455–61.

115. Ribeiro MJ, De Lonlay P, Delzescaux T, et al. Characterization of hyperinsulinism in infancy assessed with PET and 18F-fluoro-L-dopa. J Nucl Med 2005; 46(4):560–6.

116. Barthlen W, Blankenstein O, Mau H, et al. Evaluation of [18F]fluoro-L-dopa positron emission tomography-computed tomography for surgery in focal congenital hyperinsulinism. J Clin Endocrinol Metab 2008;93(3):869–75.

117. Bax KN, van der Zee DC. The laparoscopic approach toward hyperinsulinism in children. Semin Pediatr Surg 2007;16(4):245–51.

118. Fekete CN, de Lonlay P, Jaubert F, et al. The surgical management of congenital hyperinsulinemic hypoglycemia in infancy. J Pediatr Surg 2004; 39(3):267–9.

119. Filler RM, Weinberg MJ, Cutz E, et al. Current status of pancreatectomy for persistent idiopathic neonatal hypoglycemia due to islet cell dysplasia. Prog Pediatr Surg 1991;26:60–75.

120. Lee JJ, Jin CM, Kim YK, et al. Effects of anonaine on dopamine biosynthesis and L-dopa-induced cytotoxicity in PC12 cells. Molecules 2008;13(2): 475–87.

121. Lindstrom P. Aromatic-L-amino-acid decarboxylase activity in mouse pancreatic islets. Biochim Biophys Acta 1986;884(2):276–81.

122. Borelli MI, Villar MJ, Orezzoli A, et al. Presence of dopa decarboxylase and its localisation in adult rat pancreatic islet cells. Diabetes Metab 1997; 23(2):161–3.

123. Wu W, Shang J, Feng Y, et al. Identification of glucose-dependant insulin secretion targets in pancreatic beta cells by combining defined-mechanism compound library screening and siRNA gene silencing. J Biomol Screen 2008; 13(2):128–34.

124. Ribeiro MJ, Boddaert N, Bellanne-Chantelot C, et al. The added value of [18F]fluoro-L-dopa PET in the diagnosis of hyperinsulinism of infancy: a retrospective study involving 49 children. Eur J Nucl Med Mol Imaging 2007;34(12): 2120–8.

125. Otonkoski T, Nanto-Salonen K, Seppanen M, et al. Noninvasive diagnosis of focal hyperinsulinism of infancy with [18F]-dopa positron emission tomography. Diabetes 2006;55(1):13–8.

126. Subramaniam RM, Karantanis D, Peller PJ. [18F]Fluoro-L-dopa PET/CT in congenital hyperinsulinism. J Comput Assist Tomogr 2007;31(5): 770–2.

127. Mohnike K, Blankenstein O, Christesen HT, et al. Proposal for a standardized protocol for 18F-dopa-PET (PET/CT) in congenital hyperinsulinism. Horm Res 2006;66(1):40–2.

128. Hardy OT, Hernandez-Pampaloni M, Saffer JR, et al. Accuracy of [18F]fluorodopa positron emission tomography for diagnosing and localizing focal congenital hyperinsulinism. J Clin Endocrinol Metab 2007;92(12):4706–11.

129. Stanley CA, Thornton PS, Ganguly A, et al. Preoperative evaluation of infants with focal or diffuse congenital hyperinsulinism by intravenous acute insulin response tests and selective pancreatic arterial calcium stimulation. J Clin Endocrinol Metab 2004;89(1):288–96.

130. Brenner DJ, Elliston CD, Hall EJ, et al. Estimates of the cancer risks from pediatric CT radiation are not merely theoretical: comment on "Point/counterpoint: in x-ray computed tomography, technique factors should be selected appropriate to patient size: against the proposition." Med Phys 2001; 28(11):2387–8.

131. Paterson A, Frush DP. Dose reduction in paediatric MDCT: general principles. Clin Radiol 2007;62(6): 507–17.

132. Shah NB, Platt SL. ALARA: is there a cause for alarm? Reducing radiation risks from computed tomography scanning in children. Curr Opin Pediatr 2008;20(3):243–7.

133. An YS, Sheen SS, Oh YJ, et al. Nonionic intravenous contrast agent does not cause clinically significant artifacts to 18F-FDG PET/CT in patients with lung cancer. Ann Nucl Med 2007;21(10):585–92.

134. Dizendorf EV, Treyer V, Von Schulthess GK, et al. Application of oral contrast media in coregistered positron emission tomography-CT. AJR Am J Roentgenol 2002;179(2):477–81.

135. Nehmeh SA, Erdi YE, Kalaigian H, et al. Correction for oral contrast artifacts in CT attenuation-corrected PET images obtained by combined PET/CT. J Nucl Med 2003;44(12):1940–4.

136. Visvikis D, Costa DC, Croasdale I, et al. CT-based attenuation correction in the calculation of semiquantitative indices of [18F]FDG uptake in PET. Eur J Nucl Med Mol Imaging 2003;30(3):344–53.

137. Yeung HW, Sanches A, Squire OD, et al. Standardized uptake value in pediatric patients: an investigation to determine the optimum measurement parameter. Eur J Nucl Med Mol Imaging 2002; 29(1):61–6.

138. Juweid ME, Stroobants S, Hoekstra OS, et al. Use of positron emission tomography for response assessment of lymphoma: consensus of the Imaging Subcommittee of International Harmonization Project in Lymphoma. J Clin Oncol 2007;25(5):571–8.

139. Altamirano J, Esparza JR, de la Garza Salazar J, et al. Staging, response to therapy, and restaging of lymphomas with 18F-FDG PET. Arch Med Res 2008;39(1):69–77.

140. Naumann R, Vaic A, Beuthien-Baumann B, et al. Prognostic value of positron emission tomography in the evaluation of post-treatment residual mass in patients with Hodgkin's disease and non-Hodgkin's lymphoma. Br J Haematol 2001;115(4): 793–800.

Index

Note: Page numbers of article titles are in **boldface** type.

A

Aging, of gastrointestinal tract, **123–134**

B

Barium sulfate, for gastrointestinal cancer, 116
Biliary tract
    aging effects on, 129–131
    cancer of, **169–186**
        cholangiocarcinoma, 177–182
        hepatocellular carcinoma, 169–177
    normal variants of, 129–131
Biogenic amines, radiopharmaceuticals binding to,
    199
Brown fat, in esophagus, 124

C

Cancer
    gastrointestinal. *See* Gastrointestinal tract, cancer
        of; *specific locations.*
    metastatic. *See* Metastasis.
Carbon-11 acetate
    for hepatocellular carcinoma, 175, 177
    for pancreatic cancer, 159
Carbon-11 epinephrine, for neuroendocrine tumors,
    199
Carbon-11 hydroxyephedrine, for neuroendocrine
    tumors, 199, 202
Carcinoma
    cholangiocarcinoma, 177–182
    hepatocellular, 169–177, 231
Catecholamines, radiopharmaceuticals binding to, 199
Cholangiocarcinoma, 177–182
    fluorodeoxyglucose for, 178–182
    intraductal-growing, 181
    mass-forming, 180
    periductal-infiltrating, 180–181
    prognosis for, 182
    staging of, 181–182
Cholangiopancreatography, in pancreatic cancer,
    156
Colon
    aging effects on, 127–129
    cancer of. *See* Colorectal cancer.
    normal variants of, 127–129
Colorectal cancer
    in pediatric patients, 228
    metastasis from, 148–151
    PET and PET/CT in, **147–153,** 222–224
        incidental hot spots in, 148

practical considerations in, 147–148
    recurrent, 149–151
    risk stratification, 151
    staging of, 148–151
Computed tomography
    in lymphoma, 228
    in pancreatic cancer, 156–159
Contrast agents, for gastrointestinal cancer, 116–121

D

Diabetes mellitus, pancreas appearance in, 132
Diverticula, of colon, 128

E

Endoscopic cholangiopancreatography, in
    pancreatic cancer, 156, 158
Enteroclysis, PET/CT, 125–126
Erythrocytes, pitted, in elderly persons, 131–132
Esophagus
    aging effects on, 123–124
    cancer of, 136–141
        diagnosis of, 136–137
        incidence of, 135
        metastasis from, 139–141
        primary, 138–139
        recurrent, 141
        staging of, 135–138
        treatment response evaluation in, 218–221
    normal variants of, 123–124

F

Fatty acid metabolism, in hepatocellular carcinoma,
    175, 177
Fluorodeoxyglucose
    for colorectal cancer, 147–151, 222–224
    for esophageal cancer, 218–221
    for gallbladder cancer, 211
    for gastric cancer, 211, 221–222
    for gastrointestinal stromal tumors, 207–210
    for hepatoblastoma, 230–231
    for hepatocellular carcinoma, 170–176
    for liver metastasis, 189–193
    for neuroendocrine tumors, 199, 204
    for pancreatic cancer, 156–165, 211–212
    for pediatric patients, **227–238**
    gastrointestinal uptake of, normal variations and
        age effects on, **123–134**

PET Clin 3 (2008) 239–241
doi:10.1016/S1556-8598(08)00128-4
1556-8598/08/$ – see front matter © 2008 Elsevier Inc. All rights reserved.

Moving?

Make sure your subscription moves with you!

To notify us of your new address, find your **Clinics Account Number** (located on your mailing label above your name), and contact customer service at:

E-mail: elspcs@elsevier.com

800-654-2452 (subscribers in the U.S. & Canada)
314-453-7041 (subscribers outside of the U.S. & Canada)

Fax number: 314-523-5170

Elsevier Periodicals Customer Service
11830 Westline Industrial Drive
St. Louis, MO 63146

*To ensure uninterrupted delivery of your subscription, please notify us at least 4 weeks in advance of move.

ELSEVIER